The Cyclical Ketogenic Diet

The Cyclical Ketogenic Diet

A Healthier, Easier Way to Burn Fat with Intermittent Ketosis

Robert Santos-Prowse, MS, RD

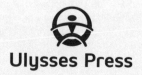

Ulysses Press

Published in the United States by:
Ulysses Press
P.O. Box 3440
Berkeley, CA 94703
www.ulyssespress.com

ISBN: 978-1-61243-869-6
Library of Congress Catalog Number: 2018959326

Printed in Canada by Marquis Book Printing
10 9 8 7 6 5 4 3 2 1

Acquisitions editor: Bridget Thoreson
Managing editor: Claire Chun
Editor: Shayna Keyles
Proofreader: Renee Rutledge
Front cover design: Chris Cote
Interior design: what!design @ whatweb.com
Cover photo: © Nina Firsova/shutterstock.com
Interior art: Geoffrey Pratt
Production: Jake Flaherty

Distributed by Publishers Group West

Contents

Preface

In my younger days, I was as clueless about nutrition as a person could be. I'd been overweight for as long as I could remember and drifted into obesity sometime around the sixth grade. I certainly made some bad choices regarding food, but I don't remember being obsessed with it or constantly eating, the way obese people are often portrayed in media. I just grew up in the toxic food environment that has existed in this country since the late 1970s.

The first edition of our government's sweeping dietary recommendations, the Dietary Guidelines for Americans, was released the same year that I was born. My weight increase followed the same trend line as the countrywide weight increase. From 1980 to 2000, the prevalence of obesity in America increased by nearly 150 percent in children and adults.

My diet was what we call the Standard American Diet, appropriately abbreviated SAD—a diet of foods that are high fat, high protein, high carbohydrate, and highly processed, such as low-quality restaurant and convenience foods. My lifestyle habits were not ideal, either. My usual after-school activity involved video games either with friends or alone. The combination of 7 hours of school and 7 or 8 hours of video games meant 14 to 15 hours of sitting almost every day. No wonder I struggled. However, it was also very frustrating because I was the only obese kid in my tight group of five or six friends. Though they were a little more reasonable than I was regarding their diet, it wasn't by much. One of them lived almost exclusively on buttered noodles and Little Debbie fudge rounds.

I occasionally tried to lose weight without much success. When I went to college, things got a little better. I was working and attending school full time, so I had far less time to sit, snack, and play video games. I lost about 20 pounds and kept it off while I completed my degree in mass communications.

After working in the print industry for a few years, I got laid off during the economic downturn of 2008-2009. I spent about 6 months looking for work without success. Then my step-father became seriously ill. He spent 11 days in the hospital and, being unemployed, I was able to spend most of that time with him. I was still obese, but my eating habits had gotten a little better.

The selections of foods offered both in the patients' rooms and in the cafeteria were appalling to me: prepackaged pastries, heat lamp-shriveled pizza, and other processed, shelf-stable crap. Even then, I had an intuitive understanding that something was wrong when a hospital, a place that is ostensibly designed with health in mind, was offering such low-quality foods.

I thought, "We have to be able to do better than this," and decided to go back to school and become a dietitian. It took me just under 5 years to complete a second undergraduate degree in human nutrition, a master's degree in clinical nutrition, and the required 1200-hour internship to become a registered dietitian. Coursework for dietitians includes a foundation in the basic sciences like chemistry, biology, physiology, and statistics, as well as a wide variety of topics related to nutrition, such as food science, psychology, and classes regarding how the body's nutritional requirements change in certain disease states.

We were taught the overly simplistic model of weight control: calories in vs. calories out. The explanation goes that weight control and fat accumulation is based purely on how much energy you put into your body vs. how much energy you use. While I had lost more weight by eating less and moving more, it was only about another 30 pounds. I was still clinically obese and being told that the answer was as simple as "eat less" was very frustrating to hear repeatedly.

We were first introduced to ketosis and a ketogenic diet during our discussions of epilepsy. For most of its history, the ketogenic diet's main use in clinical practice has been the control of epileptic seizures in children when drug therapy has been ineffective. Following accounts of fasting being used to treat epilepsy, physicians at Johns Hopkins hospital in the 1920s developed the ketogenic diet to mimic the physiological state of fasting while still being able to provide nutrition. Amazingly, as many as 90 percent of children following a therapeutic ketogenic diet report a significant reduction in the number of monthly seizures they suffer.

Other than that, the ketogenic diet was not really discussed again in my coursework. We did, however, discuss the pathways and mechanisms behind the metabolism of nutrients. We discussed how the body breaks down each of the macronutrients—carbohydrate, protein, and fat—for energy, from the mouth all the way down to the cellular level. My nutritional biochemistry professor referred to this as "energy accounting" because he would make a balance sheet for energy used versus energy produced by each process. At that time, I remember thinking that the relative metabolic inefficiency of fat and protein could be exploited for weight loss in some way, but I never made the connection with the ketogenic diet.

Later, in my graduate work, I was researching a presentation about the traditional practice of fasting during the Islamic holy month of Ramadan and kept reading about the improvement in metabolic markers like insulin sensitivity and blood glucose control during the fasting period. In addition to the measurable benefits of fasting, I read reports of increased mental clarity and higher energy levels during the fast.

I experimented with different styles of eating during my schooling. I tried vegetarian and vegan diets, a three-day "juice fast," counted carbohydrate grams using the method recommended for diabetics, and even followed the "low residue" recommendations for people who have just had surgery on their digestive system. I wanted to understand and experience what I would be recommending to people when I began to practice. This experimentation mindset eventually led to the ketogenic diet. I first tried it for myself in January 2015.

It was amazing. Once I got into ketosis, I felt incredible. I had more energy than I could ever remember, I was eating rich, delicious foods, and I lost 30 pounds over about 4 months. At the time of this writing, I have been a practicing dietitian for roughly 3 years and have been following a ketogenic diet for most of that time. I have played around with intermittent fasting, time-restricted feeding, full fasting, and, while researching this book, a cyclical ketogenic diet. I find all of them to be powerful tools with different purposes and applications.

I constantly seek out new information in the realms of diet and wellness and the more I learn, the more questions I have. Unfortunately, the science of nutrition is young and very murky. Much of the mainstream nutrition canon is based on poorly conducted science and many of the recommendations are overreaching at best. In addition to weak science, the nutrition field is plagued with bias.

There are many powerful interests at play in the Western world that stand to profit from keeping us confused. The weight-loss industry alone was valued at 68 billion dollars in 2017. We have evidence that the sugar industry, specifically the Sugar Research Foundation, withheld evidence in 1958 that linked sucrose (table sugar) to heart disease and certain types of cancer. The sugar industry was valued at 150 billion dollars in 2017. In 2015, the makers of the insulin analog Lantus, used in the management of diabetes, reported almost 7 billion dollars in sales on that drug alone. I'm not proposing a vast conspiracy. I am saying that a lot of people make a lot of money every year because what we eat is making us sick. The unfortunate truth is that we don't know nearly as much about nutrition and health as we claim to know, and what we think we know may have been influenced by forces with interests other than health.

I said in my last book that there is no one diet for everyone, but I'll take it further now: There is no one diet for everyone and everyone should follow different diet patterns at different times in their lives. You must match an eating pattern to your current goals and metabolic health. It's easier to think of your wellness needs as an equation that can be solved, but just as everything else changes in a life, so does your body, your environment, and your needs. Rather than an equation, it's more like an ongoing commitment to yourself to seek as much agency as possible over your health when there are numerous, often negative, influences at work.

Introduction

In this book, I recommend two phases of a tweaked version of a ketogenic diet. Both involve cycling in and out of ketosis on a regular basis and both, I will argue, can help you improve metabolic health, change your body composition, lose weight, supercharge cognition and focus, possibly improve athletic performance, and just plain feel awesome.

I know, I know—another diet book claiming that if you follow the author's recommendations, you'll feel like a superhero, get the body you've always wanted, and blah, blah, blah. I understand if you're skeptical. There are already a ridiculous number of books about diet and lifestyle to choose from: the Atkins diet, the South Beach diet, Whole 30, Paleo, the Zone diet, the Mediterranean diet, the Ketogenic diet, the Ketogenic Mediterranean diet (I wrote a book on that one), etc. Here's the thing, though: The SAD is so bad and so toxic that almost any intentional diet plan based on whole foods is going to be an improvement and lead to positive health outcomes. In my view, it is good that many options exist other than the default— especially if they share common themes that all point you in a direction of a lower sugar, real food-based diet. Different things resonate with each of us and we all have different psychological triggers. Perhaps, for whatever reason, reading this book will be the tipping point for you to make real change in your life.

So let's talk a little bit about the problem. America's food system and official recommendations about health and nutrition have some serious issues. More than two thirds of adults are now overweight or obese, and one out of every five children are obese. The number of individuals diagnosed with diabetes (particularly type II) has been rising consistently over the past 40 years. The American Diabetes Association estimated that the cost of care associated with diagnosed cases of diabetes was a staggering 327 billion dollars in 2017.

Of course, there are many factors contributing to the debilitating decline in our nation's (and, increasingly, the world's) health, and we can't fix everything by changing our diets and making lifestyle modifications. But many of the chronic issues we are facing can be avoided with diet and lifestyle modification, and many diseases can be, to some degree, mitigated. The body is an integrated system and giving it the appropriate fuel, physical stimulus, and recovery time better enables it to handle assaults on that system. Think of your diet and lifestyle as the foundation that the rest of your health is built upon. If the foundation is weak, the system will fail.

How to Use This Book

This book is intended for anyone looking to make a positive change in their life. It will not be highly technical but will provide sources for any relevant claims so that you can dig deeper if you get curious. (You can visit www.robertsantos prowse.com/CKD/reference for a full list of citations.)

If you have never tried a ketogenic diet but are curious, this book is for you. If you've dabbled with carbohydrate restriction but felt like it didn't work for you, keep reading. If you, like me, listen to every podcast about nutrition or health you can find, read primary research papers for fun, and regularly perform experiments on yourself to find out what makes you feel best, maybe give someone you love a nice gift of a new book. While I hope there will be some nuggets of new information for just about everyone, this book is not for the person already well on their way to optimal wellness. I intend it to be more of a starting place.

In this book, there will be quite a lot about ketosis and why you may want to cycle in and out of that state. However, we're going to start with some basic physiology and nutrition topics. I think you need a basic understanding of your body and the food you're giving it to find a diet plan that works for you long term.

After your nutrition 101 course, we'll jump right in to ketones and ketosis. I'll do my best to ensure you've got a basic understanding of what is happening in your body during ketosis, then we'll move on to discussing the two phases of the cyclical ketogenic diet. The first involves eating a very low-carbohydrate diet most of the time, with occasional forays into a moderately low-carbohydrate diet and some infrequent indulgences. The second style allows more carbohydrates more often, with occasional forays into ketosis. Both require some work and understanding of food and your body, both require quite a bit of cooking, and both will yield profound improvements in your body composition and day-to-day life.

Don't worry. I won't ask you to put in the work without preparation. In Chapters 4 and 5, you'll find sample one-week meal plans for each of the two styles, and enough recipes in Chapter 7 to get you through those weeks. Some of the recipes are simple and take only about 5 minutes; others require more prep and finesse. You decide your comfort level in the kitchen and choose accordingly. And when you just don't have the time or desire to cook, I'll try to help you navigate eating out on a ketogenic diet.

Even with the recipes, meal plans, guidance, and tips I'll give you throughout this book, your life and your diet are ultimately just that: yours. Everything in this book will require some individualization to make it right for you. Not only are all our lives different in terms of circumstance, but our individual physiologies are different as well. They're different enough that I spend Chapter 3 discussing the importance of individualization. You will have to spend some time testing these recommendations for yourself.

Even though this book is ostensibly a book about food and eating, I can't talk about diet without including other lifestyle factors. Your body processes the foods you put in it differently based on the rest of your lifestyle. Some of the benefits of lifestyle choices are obvious. If you participate in activities that build lean muscle mass, you will have positive body composition changes. Having more muscle mass increases the amount of energy you burn at rest, but it also changes what your body does with the energy it is given. Other factors that change how your body responds to food are tobacco use, sleep quality and quantity, stress factors, and, believe it or not, light exposure. To that end, Chapter 6 is dedicated to what I consider essential lifestyle considerations.

Chapter One

Basic Nutrition

To say that nutrition is basic in any way is a bit silly. Our bodies are ludicrously complicated machines with millions (if not billions) of chemical processes happening from moment to moment, and each one depends upon nutrition. Then, of course, there are the long-term consequences of what we choose to put into our body. This chapter will cover both what food actually is and what the body does with food after it is eaten.

What We're Working With

Your digestive system is basically a long tube—it has been measured at 30 feet. Each bit of the tube performs specific functions related to digestion and immunity. It starts with your mouth, ends with your anus, and has some squiggly bits in between. Those squiggly bits are your intestines and are responsible for most of the extraordinary length of the system. The small intestine alone is roughly 20 feet long.

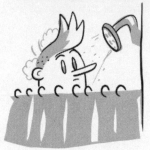

"IF THE DIGESTIVE SYSTEM IS JUST A LONG TUBE, WHEN PEOPLE KISS ARE THEY MAKING ONE REALLY LONG TUBE?"

The mouth starts the process of digestion with mechanical breakdown and lubrication of food. When you chew, you are mushing food into smaller pieces and mixing it up with your saliva, which contains enzymes to start the chemical breakdown process. Amazingly, we start the chemical breakdown of carbohydrate in the mouth. There are glands in the mouth that secrete enzymes specific to carbohydrate. That's why the longer you chew a piece of bread—even venerated whole grain bread—the sweeter it tastes.

After the mushing and enzyme action in the mouth, you swallow, and your bite of tasty whatever is pushed down the esophagus. Not much happens here except a rhythmic pushing toward the stomach called peristalsis. Your esophagus is more or less just a tube of muscle that flexes in a wave-like rhythm toward your stomach. It works even if you are upside down. Should you ever need to eat upside down, now you know that you can.

Your stomach is where the majority of breakdown happens. This is because your stomach is a bag of muscle that's full of acid. Here, fats, proteins, and carbohydrates are chemically reduced to smaller bits, sloshed around, and mixed up with enzymes and other secretions to make them ready for absorption in the small intestine. By the time it leaves the stomach, whatever you ate is now a pretty moist paste. It squirts out of a valve at the bottom of the stomach little by little as your small intestine sends signals indicating that it is ready for more.

More digestion happens in the small intestine; this is where almost all the absorption of nutrients takes place, too. Some occurs in the mouth and in the stomach, but the small intestine is where the cool stuff happens. Its internal surface is covered in tiny finger-like projections called villi that are themselves covered in even tinier finger-like projections called microvilli. There are receptors all along the villi and microvilli that react to certain nutrients, a molecule at a time. When one of those nutrients bumps into one of those receptors, it gets pulled through the wall the small intestine into the bloodstream.

After your body grabs up anything it thinks it can use, your food finally moves to the large intestine. Dangling off the area where the large and small intestines meet is a little pouch called the appendix. Many of us probably think that all the appendix does is get inflamed, explode, and kill us. As it turns out, the appendix is good for a lot more than suicide bombing. Researchers now believe that the appendix may serve as a gut flora backup of sorts. It is thought to house a collection of beneficial bacteria that can be used to reseed the gut in the event of infection, diarrhea, or other flora-compromising events like antibiotic exposure.

For many years, the large intestine was only given credit for being where poop is formed. While it is true that this is where we make poop, there is a lot more going on in the large intestine. This is where much of the microbiome is found. The microbiome is a collection of bacteria that live in our gut and are believed to have effects on everything from hunger cues to the regulation of gene expression.

The effect of the ketogenic diet on the composition of the gut microbiome in healthy individuals has not been studied very well yet. Several papers have been published showing changes to the composition of the microbiome in people using the ketogenic diet to treat certain disease states, but the value of those changes is not yet known.

While the remnants of your food make their way through the large intestine toward the exit, the bacteria eat anything they can, releasing all kinds of things as metabolic byproducts. Some of the things they produce are the nasty gasses we associate with *that end* of the body, but others are beneficial compounds like short-chain fatty acids and the protective compound butyrate. And once the food remnants reach the end of the large intestine, well, you know what happens.

What We Eat

It is incredible that we are literally made of what our parents ate and what we now eat. Our bodies take the food and non-food (like Twizzlers) that we put into it, break it down to its most basic components, and then put it back together in a wide variety of combinations. All our easily identifiable body parts, like skin and teeth and pimples, are made from the foods we choose to eat, but so are the less obvious parts of the body, like hormones and cofactors for chemical reactions. In a way,

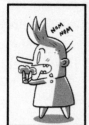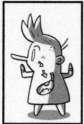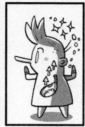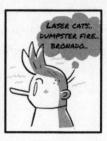

even our thoughts are made from the foods we choose to eat. Every thought we have requires both chemical energy and a variety of neurotransmitters. Guess where the chemical energy and building blocks for those neurotransmitters comes from? Yup, food.

All that is to say: What we choose to eat is important in every way in our everyday lives. Much more important than how it tastes or how we think it will affect our weight. Food can be categorized in a lot of different ways, but for the sake of this discussion, we'll keep it to macronutrients and micronutrients.

Macronutrients

Broadly speaking, the term macronutrient refers to the parts of food that the body requires in relatively large quantities to provide energy. The three main macronutrients are protein, fat, and carbohydrate.

Protein

Most of our body's tissues contain a good deal of protein, and all of our hormones and neurotransmitters require protein. Food sources of protein include all varieties of meat, eggs, most forms of dairy, nuts, seeds, and legumes, as well as some vegetables.

Protein is made of chains of molecules known as amino acids. There are many amino acids in the body at any given time, but only about 20 amino acids are worth discussing. These amino acids are the ones that the body uses to build most of our tissues, hormones, and neurotransmitters.

Of those approximately 20 amino acids, nine are considered to be essential. In this context, essential means that the body cannot synthesize them from other structures and they need to be regularly replenished through your diet. Not getting adequate amounts of these nine amino acids in your diet can lead to all sorts of nasty health outcomes from the subtle to the disastrous. The body's first response to a deficiency of essential amino acids is to break down muscle tissue to recycle some of the amino acids in that muscle.

This idea of essential amino acids is why you sometimes hear things referred to as "complete proteins." A complete protein contains all nine essentials. Many plant sources of protein do not contain all the nine essentials in sufficient amounts, which is why vegetarians are recommended to eat a variety of protein sources. It is theoretically possible, though not likely, for vegetarians to develop deficiencies if they do not eat a variety of foods.

Many protein-rich foods are also fat-rich and very beneficial to include in a ketogenic or low-carbohydrate diet. However, protein is a hotly debated topic in the keto world. The body can use some of the parts of protein to make glucose in a process called gluconeogenesis. We'll talk about all that later.

Fat

Similar to protein, fat is used in many of the body's structures, hormones, and neurotransmitters. In fact, most of the stuff in the body is made up of fat, protein, and various vitamins and minerals. Also like protein, fats are made up of chains of molecules. These chains are called fatty acids.

There are also essential and non-essential fatty acids. There are only two fatty acids that we know to be essential: linolenic and alpha-linolenic acids. Deficiencies of either can lead to skin, blood, and brain problems, though it is quite rare for adults to have diets deficient in these essential fatty acids.

Fats are generally divided into two categories: saturated and unsaturated.

SATURATED FAT

The terms saturated and unsaturated are chemistry terms. All fats are long chains of carbon molecules connected with varying amounts of hydrogen molecules tacked on. To be saturated simply means that the carbon backbone of a fat has all the hydrogen molecules it can possibly hold; it is covered to the point of saturation. These types of fats are very stable and are often solid at room temperature. Things like butter, lard, and coconut oil tend to have a greater proportion of saturated fat.

Saturated fat has been much maligned over the past several decades as the primary driver of heart disease (along with its dastardly partner, cholesterol). The thinking was that saturated fat intake increased levels of what was thought to be bad cholesterol in the blood, leading to more opportunity for bad cholesterol to build up along the walls of your arteries and eventually lead to a heart attack. This view is still maintained by much of the dominant health establishment.

However, in recent years this view has become increasingly controversial. Increasing numbers of health professionals are beginning to question the evidence used to back up the idea that dietary saturated fat increases the risk of heart disease.

There has been a push for a better analysis of the evidence, and better evidence in general. While it is possible that saturated fat intake has an impact on long-term heart health, that idea is at best overly simplistic and at worst incorrect.

UNSATURATED FAT

Unsaturated fat gets its name because it is not completely saturated with hydrogen. There are double bonds in the carbon chain at any point that is not completely saturated with hydrogen atoms. Double bonds can occur at one or more spots along the carbon backbone of a fatty acid. This is where the designations "mono" and "poly" unsaturated fat come from: Monounsaturated fats have only one spot of unsaturation, while polyunsaturated fats have more than one. Polyunsaturated fats are named based upon where along the chain the first unsaturated carbon is located. For example, omega-6 fats have their first unsaturation point at the sixth carbon along the chain, while omega-3 fats have their first unsaturation point at the third carbon along the chain.

But chemical nomenclature is not why you are reading this book. Let's move on to the food sources and possible health implications of mono- and polyunsaturated fats.

Monounsaturated fats. Monounsaturated fats are a bit of a unicorn in the food world. Though it has been included under the misguided umbrella recommendation to limit all fats, monounsaturated fat has not been singled out as a bad actor. Impressive, as almost every other food component has at one time been accused of causing ill health.

These fats are found in the greatest concentration in plant foods like olives and nuts. However, they are not exclusively found in plants. The fat in butter is, depending on the source, about a quarter monounsaturated. That's actually an important point: All fat sources are a mixture of types. The fat in olive oil, which is typically thought of as a monounsaturated fat, is only about 75 percent monounsaturated.

Foods that are primarily monounsaturated fats, like olive oils, are usually liquid at room temperature and are less shelf stable than other types of fats. That's why you need to store high-quality olive oils away from light and temperature extremes and why you should not use them to cook at high temperatures. When they are exposed to high temperatures or prolonged light, they can become rancid.

Polyunsaturated fats. There are two main types of polyunsaturated fats: omega-3 and omega-6. The distinction is important because the ratio of omega-3 to omega-6 in our diet appears to have health implications. It is thought that humans likely evolved eating a 1:1 ratio of omega-6 to omega-3 fats. However, it is estimated that people eating a Standard American Diet are likely eating a 15:1 ratio of omega-6 to omega-3. Some estimates place it as high as 25:1. It is thought that this disproportionate consumption causes higher levels of systemic and chronic inflammation, which leads to chronic disease.

Omega-6 fats are found in high concentrations in nut and seed oils and the processed foods that utilize vegetable oils.

Omega-3 fats are found in high concentrations in seafood and some types of nuts and seeds. However, the body can use the type of omega-3 fats in seafood more easily than the type found in plant sources.

Trans fats. Just like the other types of fats we've discussed so far, trans fats are named for their chemical structure. When bonds occur in chemistry, they can be either cis or trans. Those terms are directional: Cis means the bond occurs on one side, trans means the bond occurs on the other side. Though small amounts of trans fats do occur naturally in some animal products, they are typically not found in high enough concentrations to merit discussion, and they may act differently in the body. Most dietary trans fats are artificial.

Artificial trans fats are created when unsaturated fats are flooded with hydrogen to add saturation points. All you really need to know about these is that they are found exclusively in processed foods, they are associated with negative health outcomes, and the Food and Drug Administration (FDA) banned them in 2015. Of course, in true FDA fashion, they allowed until 2018 for the ban to take full effect. In short, avoid artificial trans fats whenever you can.

Cholesterol

Here, I'm referring to dietary cholesterol and not serum cholesterol. Cholesterol is a waxy fat that is found in all animal cells. Evidence suggests that for about two thirds of the population, the cholesterol that you eat has little to do with the cholesterol in your blood because your blood levels of cholesterol are determined by a complex host of other factors that are hormonally regulated. When you eat more cholesterol, your body appears to make less cholesterol. You don't need to understand much about dietary cholesterol except that the hand-wringing about eating too much of it is overblown and outdated.

Carbohydrate

Unlike protein and fat, there is no designation for any type of essential carbohydrate. Carbohydrate's main function in the body is fuel. It serves as fuel for our cells in the form of simple sugars like glucose and fructose and fuel for the bacteria in our guts in the form of non-digestible fiber.

Like protein and fat, carbohydrates are made up of long chains of molecules. In general, you should eat carbohydrates that are more difficult for your body to process and take more time to get into your bloodstream. That means you should eat carbohydrates that have been minimally processed and have high amounts of fiber. You should be getting most of your dietary carbohydrate from vegetables.

The other focal point for carbohydrate consumption is fiber. Fiber is the portion of a food that the body cannot digest and will pass through the digestive system unaltered. This is most of what the microbes in our gut use for fuel. (Fiber is also important to understand because of the idea of "net carbohydrates," which we will get into later.) There are two primary types of fiber: soluble and insoluble. The distinction just means that one forms kind of a gel and the other does not. You need both types to keep your gut happy.

Micronutrients

The micronutrients are more numerous and complicated than macronutrients. The term refers to vitamins and minerals, which are used in the countless chemical reactions taking place constantly in our bodies. While we need much less of each type of micronutrient compared to macronutrients, there are many that we cannot live well without. All the vitamins and minerals are required in some amount for optimal health, and a deficiency in any of them can have stark health consequences. The best strategy for ensuring that all your vitamin and mineral needs are met is to eat a wide variety of minimally processed foods. Just to make sure we're on the same page about what minimally processed means, I'm referring to fruits and vegetables that either start fresh or were flash frozen with no sauces or additives, meat that has had as little done to it as possible, and packaged food with very few ingredients. Now let's briefly cover the known vitamins and minerals required for health.

Vitamins

Vitamins are generally divided into two categories based on, of all things, whether they dissolve in water or fat. Therefore, the two categories are water-soluble and fat-soluble.

WATER-SOLUBLE VITAMINS

- Ascorbic Acid (C)
- Biotin (B7)
- Cobalamin (B12)
- Folic Acid (B9)
- Niacin (B3)
- Pantothenic Acid (B5)
- Pyridoxine (B6)
- Riboflavin (B2)
- Thiamin (B1)

FAT-SOLUBLE VITAMINS

- Vitamin A
- Vitamin E
- Vitamin K

For reasons I don't understand, we also call a group of hormones "vitamin D." It is considered one of the fat-soluble vitamins.

Minerals

Minerals are categorized by how much we need and how much is found in our bodies. The terms are major and trace. Minerals act as cofactors in chemical reactions but they also get directly incorporated into the body's structure. Think bones and teeth, which have high levels of calcium and phosphorus.

MAJOR MINERALS

- Calcium
- Chlorine
- Magnesium
- Phosphorus
- Potassium
- Sodium
- Sulfur

TRACE MINERALS

- Chromium
- Copper
- Fluoride
- Iodine
- Iron
- Manganese
- Molybdenum
- Selenium
- Zinc

Main Takeaways

Thanks for sticking with me this far, because
I know you did not anticipate an anatomy
and basic nutrition lesson when you picked
up this book.

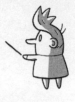

1. We are, quite literally, made of what we eat. We need
to eat a variety of the right things to function optimally.

2. The breakdown and assimilation of foods is a
complicated and nuanced process.

3. Fat and protein are essential in fairly large quantities.
Carbohydrate, less so.

4. There are a large number of micronutrients we need
to eat regularly and the best way to do that is by eating
a variety of minimally processed foods.

Chapter Two

Ketones and the Ketogenic Diet

Before we get into what a cyclical ketogenic diet looks like, we need to define ketones, ketosis, and a ketogenic diet. I believe there is a lot of confusion in the popular media related to what these terms mean and I want to make sure we're on the same page about them before moving forward.

Ketones

When you see or hear someone use the term ketones, they are almost always referring to the three molecules acetate, acetoacetate, and betahydroxybutyrate (BHB). Also, the term "ketone bodies" means the same thing. You certainly don't need to memorize these three molecules, but if you ever decided to do a deep dive into ketosis, they will come up. What is important to understand about them is that they are made in the body when fat is broken down and they can be used for fuel in almost every cell in the body. Newer research indicates that ketones are also signaling molecules and may have the effect of turning certain genes on or off.

If the body does not have adequate glucose to meet its energy needs, it will begin to break down fat instead. Fat is broken down in the liver. One of the byproducts of this process are the three ketones we mentioned above. Ironically, the liver lacks one of the enzymes needed to use ketones as fuel. So, the ketones are shuttled out of the liver, into the bloodstream, and to other cells in the body that can use them for fuel.

Most of the body's cells are able to use a combination of glucose or ketones for energy because of the cellular power plant, the mitochondria. Mitochondria are organelles found in almost every cell in the body. They produce adenosine triphosphate, which is cellular energy. Mitochondria become most efficient at using whichever fuel source they are given most often. Switching from glucose-efficient mitochondria to fat and ketone-efficient mitochondria is called mitochondrial adaptation.

Almost every system in the body can use ketones for fuel except for the red blood cell, which relies on glucose for energy. I don't want you to think that this is evidence that the body needs a steady supply of carbohydrates in the diet, though. Your body can make glucose from other sources and, since there will be some amount of carbohydrate in your diet (though not a lot), your body can allocate it to the red blood cells.

Ketosis

The term ketosis is just a shortened form of the term keto-genesis, which is made of the words "ketone" and "genesis," meaning creation. Ketosis refers to the physiological state of producing ketones in the liver. It is thought to be an evolution-ary adaptation that saves us from death by starvation when food is not available. It is the body's way of utilizing the fuel stored as fat.

When carbohydrate in the diet is absent (due to either lack of food or intentional restriction), the body will deplete the available glycogen stores first. Glycogen is the stored form of glucose. We store glycogen both in the liver and in skeletal muscle. Most people have roughly three days' worth of stored glycogen.

When all the available glycogen has been used, the body turns to fat metabolism. Our fat cells are called adipocytes and can be thought of as long-term storage centers. The process of getting fat out of the adipocytes and then converting that fat into usable energy, or ketones, is more complicated and less efficient than the process of converting and using glycogen for fuel.

Think of it like this: The food we eat is almost immediately available for use. If you're holding a sandwich, all you have to do is lift your arm and take a bite, then the energy is available. The glycogen in your liver and muscle is like the sandwich ingredients in your kitchen. They're still pretty easy to get to, prepare, and eat, but doing so requires a little more work. You've got to get up, go into the kitchen, pull all the ingredients out, and put them together before you can eat your sandwich and obtain the energy. Following this metaphor, the energy stored in your fat cells is like sandwich ingredients at the store. The energy required to obtain that sandwich is significantly higher. You've got to go to the store, select the ingredients, pay for them, come back home, then assemble your sandwich before you can even take a bite.

This metaphor illustrates the availability of fuel, as well. There is much, much more food at the store than there is stored in your refrigerator at home. Everyone, even very lean individuals, have a whole lot more energy stored as fat than they do stored as glycogen. Your glycogen storage capacity typically maxes out at about 10,000 calories, while there is no known upper limit for fat storage. Even people with very little body fat have upwards of 100,000 calories stored as fat. This is a pretty incredible system. It allows us to deal with very long periods of lack of food with relative ease. For example, a 27-year-old Scottish man weighing 456 pounds fasted under medical supervision for a full 382 days and received only vitamin and mineral supplementation in addition to non-caloric beverages. Three hundred eighty-two days! So even when you feel like you're going to die if you don't have some French fries, trust me, you're going to be okay.

After your glycogen stores have been depleted, the liver will send signals to mobilize the fat stored in your adipocytes. The fat will get dumped into your bloodstream and travel to the liver, where it is broken down for energy. During the break-down, ketones are produced as well. As I said earlier, the liver can't use ketones so it spits them back into the bloodstream to be transported and used in other organs throughout the body.

I want to take a moment to clear up a misconception I see repeated all over the keto-sphere. Ketosis is not a binary condition; it is not like a light switch that is either on or off.

Your body's energy management is dynamic and varied. Your cells will use glucose, ketones, free fatty acids, lactic acid, and a few other sources as fuel for their chemical reactions. When we say "in ketosis," what is actually meant is that the concentration of ketones is at a certain level. Nutritional ketosis is the state that you are shooting for, and it just means that your primary fuel source, at a cellular level, is fat rather than carbohydrate. Even during deep nutritional ketosis, your body is still using glucose as fuel to some degree. So it's really about fuel ratio.

Before we move on to the ketogenic diet, we have to talk briefly about ketoacidosis and the important difference between it and nutritional ketosis.

Nutritional Ketosis

This term refers to the type of ketosis we will be discussing in this book. It is the elevation of ketones in your blood due to the intentional restriction of carbohydrates in the diet. It is safe and has many metabolic advantages. Nutritional ketosis is regarded as having blood measurements of BHB in the .05 mmol to 3.5 mmol range.

Ketoacidosis

Ketoacidosis is a life-threatening condition in which blood levels of ketones reach such concentrations that your blood becomes too acidic. Ketones are very mildly acidic, so if you get a whole bunch of them in your blood at once, it can lower the pH of your blood to dangerously acidic levels. The concentration of BHB needs to be upward of 8 mmol in order for this to be an issue. This is not a situation that will happen under normal physiological conditions. That is, unless you have type

I diabetes or very advanced type II diabetes, this is not a thing you need to worry about.

You will likely, however, have to understand the difference well enough to explain it to well-meaning friends when they tell you that you are endangering your life by eating a ketogenic diet. The best way I've found to quickly get people to understand the difference is like this: Consider a nice, toasty fire in your fireplace and a house fire. The mechanism is the same in both situations but one is beneficial and contained while the other is dangerous and out of control.

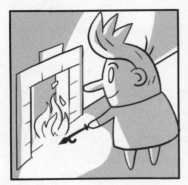 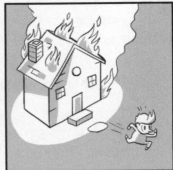

The Ketogenic Diet

So now that you know about ketones and ketosis, I bet you can guess what "ketogenic diet" means. It is just a diet that induces a state of ketosis. In its simplest form, all a ketogenic diet needs to be is a diet that contains very little carbohydrate and enough (but not too much) protein.

The classical ketogenic diet was developed in the early 1920s by physicians and researchers at Johns Hopkins University and the Mayo Clinic to treat epilepsy. They noticed that fasting seemed to have some therapeutic effect on children with epilepsy who were not responding to other treatment. They wanted to develop a diet that put the body into a state that was similar to fasting. The diet they developed was a 4:1 ratio of fat calories to protein and carbohydrate calories. This is a very strict restriction and very hard to follow. However, it works. Following this restriction will very reliably induce ketosis and offer improvements in seizure control for those suffering from epilepsy. This regimen was used heavily until the late 1930s, when anticonvulsant drugs were introduced to control epilepsy.

The ketogenic diet fell out of favor until the 1970s when Dr. Robert Atkins popularized it for weight loss with his *Dr. Atkins Diet Revolution*. Since that time, interest in the ketogenic diet has waxed and waned repeatedly but never really gone away. People follow the diet, lose weight, and feel great. Then they get tired of the restriction, afraid of all the fat, or too temped by the sea of hyper-processed carbohydrates in our food supply.

Recently, there has been a surge in interest in the ketogenic diet in both the popular media and scientific literature. According to Google's search term tracking tool, Google Trends, search volume for the term "ketogenic diet" has increased 97 percent between December 2016 and July 2018, and the trend line appears to still be heading up. Scientific research about ketones and the ketogenic diet has seen a similar explosion during the past 5 years.

Scientists are investigating many new and interesting aspects of ketosis. It has been well established for many years that a ketogenic diet can be a very effective tool for weight loss and body composition management and, as mentioned above, the control of epilepsy. We are now learning that this may only be the tip of the iceberg. Researchers are finding benefits for many disease states including Alzheimer's and other neurodegenerative diseases, almost all forms of metabolic dysfunction including diabetes and metabolic syndrome, cardiovascular disease, and cancer. In addition to the benefit that ketosis can offer us when things go wrong, research is starting to indicate that ketones themselves may change our DNA expression in ways that make us more resilient to the aging process in general.

Additionally, tons of anecdotal accounts testify to the power of the ketogenic diet. Many amazing stories of weight loss can be found, but there are also countless reports of freedom from cravings and newfound mental clarity that accompany a ketogenic diet. Many people report sharpened focus and mental acuity once they are adapted to ketosis. I myself have had this experience.

When I first approached a ketogenic diet, I did it rather haphazardly and experienced a difficult transition from glucose metabolism to fat metabolism over the course of about three days. Near the end of the third day, it was as if a switch was flipped and I suddenly went from feeling slightly worse to feeling amazingly better than I could remember. My energy level was higher and more stable, I could focus for long periods of time, and I felt just a little sharper in general. This type of thing is incredibly hard to prove with empirical data but I have heard it repeated over and over again.

Mechanistically, the increased stability of energy makes sense. We know that most of the cells in the body can use fat and ketones instead of glucose for fuel, and we know that we all have much more fat stored as energy than we do glucose. So, if we transition from a state of having to rely on a constantly diminishing glucose supply (glucose metabolism) to a state of burning fat for fuel, we are able to tap into a much larger energy reserve. The incredible sense of clarity is a little less easy to explain. Perhaps the brain likes ketones better than glucose for fuel, perhaps it is the same mechanism as the sustained energy for the rest of body, and maybe it is just a placebo effect.

The net effect of this increased interest in the ketogenic diet has been a huge increase in the body of knowledge that we have about ketosis, a host of new products available to those trying to live a low-carb lifestyle, and two book deals for me. Joking aside, just as with the surge in interest about gluten restriction a few years ago, this uptick in interest about the ketogenic diet and ketosis has been fantastic for those of us trying to adhere to a ketogenic diet. More products are available but there are also now many more options at restaurants, and the restaurants that do not have menu items specifically meant for low-carb dieters are often willing to make accommodations. Physicians, dietitians, and other health-care practitioners are also now more likely to have heard of the ketogenic diet and maybe even seen the beneficial effects of it firsthand.

The future of the ketogenic diet looks like it will be even more liberalized than it is now because there are more tools to help your body achieve ketosis than there ever have been before. There is a type of fat called medium chain triglycerides (MCT) that has been shown to promote the production of ketones. Until recently, one needed to use oils to get effective doses of MCTs, and that was problematic because many people find that MCTs can cause upset stomach or diarrhea. Now there are an abundance of MCT oil powders on the market that are also effective at raising blood ketone levels but do not appear to come with the same GI upset.

Another class of useful products that has come about in recent years is exogenous ketones. In this context, exogenous means something that comes from outside the body. There are now many brands of exogenous ketones on the market and many of them have been shown to reliably raise blood ketone levels quickly and substantially. They come as liquids and can be prohibitively expensive. The important thing to understand about exogenous ketones is that while they will raise your blood levels of ketones, they do not produce a state of ketosis. What I mean is that they don't get your body to start making ketones the way that carbohydrate restriction does. You're just literally dumping ketones into your system.

Main Takeaways

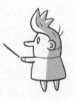

1. Ketones are the molecules that your body uses for fuel when there is not enough glucose. They are also anti-inflammatory and may be protective against some scary diseases.

2. Ketosis is the term for the state your body is in when it is making ketones. This happens when you restrict carbohydrates in the diet. It is not the same thing as ketoacidosis.

3. A ketogenic diet is a way of eating that promotes the state of ketosis. It is a very low-carbohydrate, moderate-protein, and high-fat diet. It is safe and beneficial.

Chapter Three

The Importance of Self-Knowledge

There are billions of humans on this planet. Every one of them is unique. The idea that we will all react the same way to a diet is, frankly, just bonkers. One-size-fits-all is fine for hats, but not for diet or lifestyle. Diet and lifestyle choices are either custom tailored or they don't fit.

In this chapter I am going to discuss why knowing yourself and your body is non-negotiable for success with any diet or lifestyle goal. I am not going to go so far as to recommend that you do extensive and frequent blood testing (though if that's your jam, go for it), but you absolutely need a good understanding of your body and how it reacts to different stimuli.

I will make recommendations and give you a lot of recipes, but what has worked for me may not work for you. Maybe you are a person who feels bloated and cruddy after any amount of gluten exposure. Maybe you don't tolerate dairy that well and will need to limit the amount you consume. Perhaps you are a person with the genetic variant that makes fresh cilantro taste like soap.

Even though we have a much better understanding of what's going on in the body during ketosis than we did a decade ago, there is still much we do not know. One of those things is the exact limit of carbohydrate restriction that will induce keto-genesis. Of course, it appears to vary a great deal from person to person and there are many factors that determine your partic-ular limit of carbohydrate tolerance. Some of these factors are obvious and can be measured, like amount of muscle mass and level of insulin resistance. Other factors are less obvious, like exactly how much glycogen your liver can store, what your microbiome is doing, and how good your cellular machinery is at burning fat. Some people have an incredibly easy time getting into and maintaining ketosis, while others find it to be a challenge.

Researchers at the Weizmann Institute of Science published research in 2015 showing that postprandial glucose response (how much your blood sugar rises in response to a meal) appears to be much more variable from person to person than we previously thought. The researchers gave 800 people devices that measured their blood glucose levels every 5 minutes and tracked those levels for a week. During that week, the participants were asked to record everything they ate as well as their physical activity. They were also given test meals that the researchers had specifically formulated. Strikingly, the rise in blood sugar across 795 people recorded after a standardized serving of bread was 44 ± 31 mg/dl*h (milligrams of glucose per deciliter of blood over 1 hour), with the bottom 10 percent of participants exhibiting an average increase below 15 mg/dl*h and the top 10 percent of participants exhibiting an average increase above 79 mg/dl*h. To me, that says that generalized recommendations are fuzzy guidelines at best. With that much variability between people, health authorities really can't tell you how your body is going to react to a certain food item with any amount of certainty.

I understand that it is not practical for everyone to measure their blood glucose levels every 5 minutes and create detailed spreadsheets of how different foods affect them. I just want you to understand that we are all truly unique and to achieve optimal health, we have to approach our health in a unique and individual way.

Ketosis and Your Body

In the context of a ketogenic diet, you are going to want to have a baseline understanding of your body and how well it can handle certain carbohydrate-containing foods because the main determining factor for achieving ketosis is the amount of glucose your body has available for fuel. If there are foods that you love that the conventional wisdom would advise you to restrict but, because of your particular response to them, can be included in your diet without negative consequence, wouldn't you want to know? If you're anything like me, you're going to want to know roughly how much carbohydrate you can have in a day before kicking yourself out of ketosis. I don't think it is possible (or desirable!) to know down to the gram, but it is nice to have a rough idea.

After you have experienced what ketosis feels like and have switched back to normal glucose metabolism a few times, you will start to be able to tell when you are in ketosis and when you are not. I can tell if I've overdone it on the carbs and knocked myself out of ketosis because I have a period of feeling sluggish and run down. If I make a series of particularly bad food decisions, I will actually feel somewhat hung over the following morning. You may or may not feel the metabolic change as acutely as I do.

In less subjective terms, there are a few ways to measure ketosis. You may find these valuable until you are comfortable judging only by feeling. There are three methods for measuring ketosis: by urine, breath, and blood.

Urine Measurement. Urine acetoacetate (remember, the three ketone bodies are acetoacetate, acetate, and betahydroxybutyrate [BHB]) levels are measured using an indicator stick that will change colors based on the concentration detected. These are cheap, readily available, and not terribly useful long term. You may find utility with them in the beginning of your experience with a ketogenic diet. They are useful for giving a binary "yes" or "no" if you are in ketosis or not.

Breath Measurement. There are now several devices on the market that will measure the level of acetoacetate in your breath. The advantage of these is that they are reusable and non-invasive. From what I've seen, they appear to be useful in broad terms. They can tell you if you are in ketosis and if you vary from day to day depending on what you eat, your activity level, your sleep, etc. They, like the urine measurement, are not all that specific in terms of how deep into ketosis you are, and they are rather expensive on the front end. Some of the devices cost several hundred dollars.

Blood Measurement. This is the gold standard for ketone measurement. It measures the amount of BHB in your circulating blood. Since BHB is the primary ketone used for fuel while in ketosis, this is the most relevant to measure. It also appears to be the most accurate and sensitive. With this form of measurement, you can really determine the effect certain foods have on your level of ketosis. This may be useful because it will allow you to get a sense of how much wiggle room you have in your daily carbohydrate intake, and it will let you know if your specific reaction to any foods is different from what the common knowledge says it should be. Of course, the downside to this type of measurement is that you have to use blood. The device used for this is a glucometer, the same as what people with diabetes use to check their blood sugar levels. They require a different type of test strip, though. There are a few on the market now and while the devices themselves are inexpensive, the test strips used can add up quickly. So, the cons of this method are that it can also be cost prohibitive and you have to stick your finger each time you want to measure.

If you choose to measure your ketone level, no matter which method you use, your goal should be to increase your self-knowledge. Be sure to note how you feel when the meter or test strip reads a certain level. If you expect it to say one thing but it comes out something else, try to think of why that may be. What did you do differently that day?

Food Allergies and Sensitivities

Though it is necessary for life and we often love putting it in our bodies, food is still a foreign substance that has to be processed by the body. Sometimes, our bodies think foods are pathogens and react by activating the immune system. It doesn't take a lot of careful attention to yourself and your feelings to know if you have a true and severe allergy. You'll notice if you suddenly can't breathe after you eat peanuts.

Food sensitivities, sometimes called intolerances, are much less obvious but are still worth discovering and managing. Common things that people report that they have issues with are cow's milk and associated products, gluten, eggs, some artificial sweeteners and dyes, nuts, and the additive MSG. I have heard from many people over the years that they feel better when not consuming one or, in some cases, all those things.

If you're not feeling great, it is worth doing some investigative work and paying attention to how you feel after eating just about everything. If you notice that you have really bad gas and sometimes diarrhea after you drink cow's milk or eat a lot of cheese at once, you're likely intolerant to some portion of dairy.

If the sensitivity is less obvious, it may require a more systematic approach to discover. Elimination diets are short-term restrictive diets that, as the name implies, eliminate all the common allergens and irritants from your diet for a short period, typically 2 weeks, and then add them back in, one at a time, so that you can determine what specific thing is causing you discomfort. You can easily find a step-by-step guide to an elimination diet on the internet if you choose to pursue one.

I know that an elimination diet sounds like a lot of trouble, but if there is something in your diet preventing you from feeling your best on a daily basis, it is absolutely worth the trouble.

Caffeine Intake

Caffeine is a stimulant that interferes with your body's natural sleep regulation system. It is worth finding out your tolerance to this common stimulant because it can be a sneaky disruptive force in your life if it is responsible for you getting less than optimal sleep.

If you have issues sleeping, the generally repeated rule of thumb for caffeine is "no caffeine after 2 p.m." While this could be a good place to start, you can always get more specific. I can drink strong coffee well into the evening and have no issue falling asleep when my day is finally done. My wife can't really have any significant source of caffeine past noon or she will have a harder time falling asleep. Our toddler can't even handle one shot of espresso in the morning! (Just kidding.)

Gender, tobacco usage, hormonal contraceptive use, and just plain old interpersonal variability all play a role in how quickly your body will clear a dose of caffeine and how acutely you will feel that dose. Just pay attention to when you have your last coffee, tea, or other caffeinated beverage of choice and how well you sleep that night. If you've got the rest of your sleep hygiene (we'll talk about that in Chapter 6) dialed in, then you know it was the caffeine messing with your sleep quality and can adjust your intake accordingly.

Understand Your Limits

You need to understand your limits to be successful with any lifestyle change. You may be ready and willing to cut out all the sweets, breads, pastas, and potatoes from your diet but can't quite handle getting rid of the fruits just yet. Knowing that may require you to transition into a ketogenic diet more slowly than someone who is ready to just jump right in. While that may feel frustrating, accepting that knowledge can set you up for success. If you take on more than you are personally ready for, you are just setting yourself up for failure.

If I tell you to cut out most of the carbohydrates from your life and start caring about food quality, sleep quality, physical activity, community participation, mindfulness, and a sense of purpose, you could understandably feel overwhelmed. Every day we make thousands of choices, and researchers believe that we actually have a finite amount of willpower each day. Every time we make a choice that requires choosing one thing over another, we are spending a little bit of that willpower—or more, if it feels like we are depriving ourselves of something. That's why some powerful and high-achieving people have taken steps to reduce the amount of decisions they have to make in a day. Notably, Barak Obama and Steve Jobs both wore more-or-less the same outfit on non-event days so that they would not have to spend any of their decision-making budget on something relatively unimportant, like clothing. It is also part of the reason that many stores are just cram-jam with stuff these days. If you have to say no to 10,000 products before getting to the register, you may be more likely to say yes to an impulse buy waiting in line. Twix bar, anyone? How about a Snickers? What about a king-sized Reese's Cup, or a Twizzlers, or some chips, or a Coke?

So pick your battles. Don't try to change too many big things too quickly. Otherwise, you'll probably find yourself thinking, "I just can't handle thinking about carbohydrates or blue light exposure harming my sleep quality. I need to eat dinner and relax." So maybe you order pizza or make yourself a sandwich. Maybe you watch some TV or play a game on your phone. Whatever you choose, instead of beating yourself up, take it as an opportunity to learn more about yourself and potentially make different choices in the future.

It is important that you are honest with yourself, too. Are you really incapable of spending any more effort today, or are you not really committed to making this change? That is an important distinction, and I can't tell you how to determine it in the moment. As with any form of self-awareness, learning this distinction takes time. You may not be in the habit of thinking critically about your quantity or quality of choices each day, and the idea of doing such a thing may seem tedious and impossible, but there are people who do it every day out of necessity. Individuals with disability are required to ration their efforts and adapt to their limitations so that they may focus on their priorities. Instead of focusing on the work of participating in this balancing act, consider that you are creating more space for joy and fulfillment.

Also, remember that making a lifestyle change is not an all-or-nothing proposition, and a failure in one area does not constitute an overall failure or mean that you should give up. It's common for people to lament over failed attempts at change, especially in a diet and lifestyle context, but it's important for us to reframe this popular narrative. In reality, changes are slow going and take sustained effort, and by giving yourself opportunities to make different choices than you have before, you're creating space for small steps toward your goals. Wayne Gretzky said, "You miss 100% of the shots you don't take." Giving yourself opportunities to make different choices is already a step in the right direction. Instead of focusing on big end-goal fantasies, look at the small steps you've taken. Just give yourself permission.

Main Takeaways

1. Everyone is different and will respond to inputs like carbohydrates, caffeine, and common food irritants differently.

2. Knowing your specific limits and tolerance levels is important for success and worth the work.

3. You have a finite amount of willpower in a day and when you "can't even" any more, you're unlikely to make the best choices for your health. Start by being realistic about your own ability and learn from your moments of burnout.

Chapter Four

The Cyclical Ketogenic Diet Phase 1:

Fat Adaptation and Weight Loss

This phase of the diet actually has two stages in itself. The first is getting you into ketosis and letting your mitochondria adapt to burning fat, and the second is keeping it up until you meet your weight-loss goals. If you are one of the rare individuals that does not have weight-loss goals, it is still important that you follow the first portion of this phase. Mitochondrial adaptation to a high-fat diet is nonnegotiable for the cyclical ketogenic diet. Even if you are only interested in the energy, cognition, and performance benefits of the ketogenic diet and do not desire to lose any body weight, do not skip this step.

Ketosis will change you in a variety of ways. It will change the choices you make, how you look, how you think about and interact with food, and your metabolism. It will even change you on a genetic level. I believe that all these changes will be positive but I also don't believe they are enough. You can technically follow a ketogenic diet in a very unhealthy and unsustainable way. I'm going to give you an outline of what to eat from a macronutrient composition lens but I'll also be discussing food quality and micronutrient considerations.

Consider Where You're Starting

Extreme carbohydrate restriction is not an easy thing to do in this day and age. It is easier than it once was but it still requires quite a lot of planning and willpower to make it work. An important consideration is your starting point and how drastic of a change a ketogenic diet will be for you. Is your baseline diet pretty low in carbohydrates already or are you a carboholic? Do you already include some fats in your diet or does your typical day follow a bagel-sandwich-pasta pattern?

I've existed at both ends of that spectrum and I've entered ketosis from both a low-carbohydrate pattern and a pretty much all-carbohydrate pattern. Let me tell you, from a subjective perspective, it is a heck of a lot easier psychologically and physiologically to transition into ketosis without negative side effects if you're already eating a low-carbohydrate diet. Psychologically, it is easier to adhere to the restriction if you've already been avoiding breads and pastas and sweets. It felt to me as though the transition from glucose metabolism to fat metabolism was seamless when I was already eating a diet pretty low in carbohydrate. As you might expect, I experienced more hunger and a bit of lightheadedness when I was eating a lot of carbohydrate prior to entering ketosis.

If you take stock of your diet and find yourself closer to the high-carbohydrate end of the spectrum, I would recommend taking a couple of weeks to gradually reduce your baseline carbohydrate intake before fully restricting to a ketogenic level. I think that this, paired with proper hydration and electrolyte management, will make the transition into ketosis very smooth. So start by avoiding concentrated and very easily digestible carbohydrates like sweets, breads and other grains, and pastas. Replace these foods with higher fat whole foods and vegetables.

For example, if you typically have a bagel, cereal, or oatmeal for breakfast, try switching these foods out for some fried or scrambled eggs with cheese and avocado or a fruit smoothie. If you typically have a sandwich, either try replacing it with a salad that has similar ingredients or just skip the bread and try it as a lettuce wrap. For dinner, instead of pizza or pasta, try having a stir-fry with protein of your choice, a bean and meat chili, or a simple meat-and-potato type of dish. If you currently snack in between your meals, it would be best for you to just break that habit. That's the eventual goal. But, if you find that to be very challenging, stick to fruit, nuts and seeds, jerky, hard-boiled eggs, and cheese.

The idea of this period is to get yourself physically and emotionally acclimated to the idea of extreme carbohydrate restriction. Once you've gotten your diet reasonably cleansed of low-quality carbohydrates, it should be easier for you to go the rest of the way to a full ketogenic diet.

Goal Setting

Before you get started with the cyclical ketogenic diet, you should take some time to consider your overall relationship with your food, your body, and your goals. Why do you want to follow a cyclical ketogenic diet? Are you trying to lose weight and change your body composition, cut your sugar cravings, break your addiction to food, get better mental clarity, or some other reason entirely? Take a moment and actually write down what you want to get from the lifestyle changes you are making. I recommend you write it down somewhere you can see it on a regular basis, like a sticky note, a mirror, or a digital note on the homepage of your phone.

If weight loss is one of your goals, as it was for me when I started giving more attention to my health, I suggest you write down two more reminders. First, you should have a scale victory, which is a number you would like to see on your scale. Second, you should give yourself a non-scale victory. This can be anything you want it to be, but it should be something concrete that will make you feel good when it happens. It could be fitting into a specific size of clothing or even a specific piece of clothing. I don't know about you, but I had clothes that I'd been keeping for years, thinking, "I'll look great in that if I lose a few more pounds." It could also be behavior related—maybe your non-scale victory has to do with choosing a more healthy coping mechanism in response to stress if emotional eating is a habit of yours.

Goal setting in this way is important because it allows you to have a victory condition that you can see and keep in your vision. Having a non-scale victory condition is important because, frankly, scales can be mean-spirited liars. All sorts of things can affect the number on a scale and you may be making very real progress that you just don't see. If you tie up too much of your esteem in that number, it is easy to become discouraged when it doesn't drop as quickly as you would like.

Stage 1—Strict Ketosis

The goal of phase 1's first stage is to get your body into ketosis and keep it there long enough for the metabolic, hormonal, and epigenetic changes necessary for efficient fat burning (referred to collectively as "fat adaptation") to take place. I want to say this up front: No one knows how long this takes and it is likely variable from person to person. The best and most generalized guess we have is that it takes 4 to 8 weeks for your body to start using fat efficiently when deprived of carbohydrate.

You may have read before that it takes 3 weeks to solidify a new habit. It turns out, like almost everything, that the truth appears to be much less uniform. Research indicates that there is a huge degree of variability between individuals in how long it takes for something to become an automatic habit. Some people took as long as 66 days to habitually do something as simple as eat a piece of fruit with breakfast. Since omitting almost all carbohydrates is much more complicated than just eating a piece of fruit with breakfast, I am going to recommend that you strictly adhere to carbohydrate (and protein) restriction for somewhere between 30 and 60 days before moving on to the next stage.

I asked Tommy Wood, MD, PhD, and the team at Nourish Balance Thrive, a health and wellness company specializing in performance and human optimization, to elaborate a bit about this adaptation stage. Dr. Wood and the folks at Nourish Balance Thrive have helped thousands of people feel great and achieve their goals over the years. Here's what they said:

> On average, 30 to 60 days is a good target for most people to become at least relatively "keto adapted," assuming we're not talking to athletes looking for performance. If you're measuring fasted morning BHB, you'd probably see an increase in the first few weeks, which then comes down to a more stable level, often between 0.5 and 1.0mmol once adapted. More importantly, though, is probably subjective symptoms. Once you're feeling good and sleeping well, you're probably keto-adapted. If you never feel good eating keto, this is a good sign that you should be looking elsewhere to improve your health.

The "elsewhere" mentioned above has to do with other lifestyle factors that we will discuss in Chapter 6: Diet Is Not Enough.

Remember, our goal here is to literally change you on a cellular level. I know that two months may seem like a really long time to follow a strict ketogenic diet but it will be worth it.

Restricting Carbohydrates

There is really only one requirement to get your body to produce ketones: deprive it of glucose. So, the ketogenic diet is all about restricting carbohydrate intake. The specific amount you need to restrict varies from person to person based on things like genetics, body composition, insulin sensitivity, and activity level. To be safe and give yourself the best shot at getting into ketosis, you should aim to eat no more than 30 grams of total carbohydrate per day until you feel that you have achieved ketosis. You can then play with that number a bit and determine if your body can handle more or if you need to restrict even further.

Let's go ahead and talk about the difference between total and net carbohydrates. Total is just what it sounds like—the total amount of carbohydrate found in a food. Net is what is left if you subtract grams of fiber, which your body cannot digest, from total carbohydrate. Some advocate for using net carbohydrate grams rather than total carbohydrate grams for your daily carbohydrate budget. The rationale is that your body cannot digest the fiber portion of food so it will not be broken down to glucose, will not raise blood glucose, and will not promote an insulin response. While this theory is technically sound, it does not come without caveats.

Depending on what you are eating, the numbers you are using for carbohydrate and fiber may not be accurate. If it is a whole food like a strawberry or avocado, there is bound to be huge variability between the nutrition information you have access to and what is in the actual foods, which do not have nutrition labels. The best information you have at your disposal is the USDA nutrient database. That's also the database that most popular food tracking apps, like MyFitnessPal, use for their nutrient information.

Think about it: the USDA data is based upon the nutritional composition of a strawberry or an avocado that was tested in a lab somewhere, not the one you are eating. There are likely many important differences between the food tested and the food you're eating, like physical size, soil quality, ripeness, farming practices, and possibly, strain of seed used. All these factors may make the information available to us about carbohydrate and fiber content incorrect to some degree.

For restaurant foods, the variability is multiplied. In addition to the issues discussed above, there's the human aspect of variability. Let's say you go to a chain restaurant and order something based on the nutrition information they provide to you. Unless the worker making your food that day uses the exact corporate prescribed amount of each ingredient for your particular food, the nutrition information you've been provided won't match the actual nutrients in your food.

Processed foods are actually likely to have the most accurate nutrition information. Because they are often made in an industrial setting using automated processes and very precise ingredient controls, it is more likely that each individual product will be similar to the test product. However, even these foods are not totally accurate. The FDA allows for up to 20 percent variability of nutrition content from what is listed on a label and does not have any verification system in place to check that what producers list is accurate.

You may be thinking, "That applies to all nutrition information, so it would apply to using total carbohydrates for my budget, too." You are absolutely correct. The issue with net carbohydrates is that you are introducing two variables so the problem has the potential to be doubled. If the total carbohydrate number on a label is less than the actual total carbohydrate in your food and the fiber number on that label is more than the actual amount of fiber in your food, well, you see the issue.

If you do choose to use net carbohydrate over total carbohydrate, you will be allowed a higher carbohydrate intake, and it may even help you to get more fiber in your diet. However, if you choose to use net carbohydrate, you should probably build some room for error into your daily carbohydrate budget.

Maybe shoot for 20 net grams if you think your actual toler-ance is 30 net grams.

Since you have such a small budget for carbohydrates per day, I recommend that you try to get the majority of them from non-starchy vegetables. Not only are those vegetables deli-cious, but they also contain valuable vitamins and minerals that you may not otherwise be able to get in your diet. As we covered in Chapter 1, there are a lot of trace minerals that you need to regularly replenish and the best way to do that is by eating a varied diet, which includes vegetables. Additionally, non-starchy vegetables are a good way to get the indigest-ible fiber that your microbiome needs to thrive. Including adequate fiber can help prevent one of the most-often cited "side effects" of a ketogenic diet: constipation. I think the cause of any constipation during a ketogenic diet is likely due to inadequate fiber intake and possibly a disrupted gut flora population. You can mitigate both of those issues by easing into a ketogenic diet as I recommended earlier and by trying to get the majority of your carbohydrate intake from vegetables.

The microbes in our guts are specialists in regard to what they digest. If you typically eat a SAD, your microbiome is going to be comprised of a lot of bacteria that enjoy that type of food—or rather, food-like products that contain a lot of easy-to-digest simple carbohydrate and highly processed and inflammatory oils. As you increase the amount of fibrous carbohydrates and reduce the amount of simple carbohydrates you are giving your gut, some of the microbes that live on the simple carbohy-drates will starve, while those that are better at digesting fiber will thrive. If you make this change too quickly, your microbi-ome population may not have adequate time to adjust and you may experience some unpleasant gastric growing pains like constipation or diarrhea, gas and bloating, and maybe some nausea. Nobody wants that.

Eating Enough Protein

Believe it or not, protein is controversial in the ketogenic community. There are two camps: one that believes you should restrict protein, and one that believes you shouldn't.

The first camp believes you should restrict protein as well as carbohydrates because your body has the capability to make glucose from protein through a process called gluconeogenesis. The thought is that once your needs for cellular repair and muscle synthesis are met, the excess protein you eat will be broken down and converted to glucose for energy. If this happens, you will no longer be in ketosis. Dr. Peter Attia, a physician, podcast host, and prominent figure in the ketosis and longevity world, has repeatedly mentioned that he can't have more than 100 to 110 grams of protein in a day or it will knock him out of ketosis for a time.

The other camp argues that while glucose and insulin levels are low (as they should be in ketosis), the body will not turn proteins into glucose at levels sufficient to interfere with ketone production, no matter how much protein you eat. Dr. Benjamin Bikman, professor of physiology and developmental biology at Brigham Young University, told me about the process:

> *Individual amino acids have varying effects on insulin secretion and, thus, have an indirect effect on ketogenesis. However, it's also true that some of these same amino acids (e.g., leucine) can be converted directly into ketones, known appropriately as "ketogenic amino acids." Nevertheless, the degree to which*

ingested protein, which is made of individual amino acids, increases insulin is dependent on underlying glucose levels. If glucose is elevated, such as in a high-carbohydrate diet, protein elicits an insulin effect (and indirectly inhibits ketogenesis). However, if glucose consumption is low, the liver is actively creating glucose to make up for what's not consumed, a process termed gluconeogenesis. This process, like ketogenesis, can only happen when insulin is low. With this in mind, it's not surprising that dietary protein has little or no effect on insulin when coupled with a low-carbohydrate diet— the body cannot afford to stop gluconeogenesis. Thus, gluconeogenesis and ketogenesis remain unimpaired.

I personally have not noticed an issue with a large intake of protein, but I've also never directly tested my blood level of BHB before and after. I've just gone by how I feel. The important thing here is that it has not been studied in a rigorous way and it is likely different for everyone. I recommend that you shoot for 1.2 to 2.0 grams of protein per kilogram of lean body mass depending on your activity level and preference. If you participate in a lot of muscle-dependent activity like resistance training, shoot for the higher end. If you don't engage your muscles very much or if you are finding it difficult to achieve nutritional ketosis, shoot for the lower end.

Probably the easiest way to determine your lean body mass is to use a bioelectric impedance device. Many bathroom scales now come equipped with the capability to measure lean body mass through the use of bioelectric impedance. You just place your feet (and, if it is a higher-end device, your hands) on metal sensors. The device runs a very mild (you don't even feel it) electric current through your body and, based upon the resistance of different types of tissue, can tell you your fat mass, bone mass, lean body mass, and hydration status. It is important to note that even the best of these devices is not terribly accurate. However, they are accurate enough for the purpose of determining your starting place for protein intake. You'll be tweaking up or down based on your personal feedback anyway.

You don't want to neglect your protein intake for several reasons. As discussed earlier, protein is needed for muscle, hormones, DNA, and just about everything else. You also don't want to undershoot the protein intake because, remember, you're working with three macronutrients—fat, protein, and carbohydrate. You're already restricting carbohydrates pretty severely. If you also practice a severe protein restriction, you're going to end up drinking olive oil to get your calories. No fun.

Eating Plenty of Fat

You're going to be eating a lot of fat on the ketogenic diet. A lot. But that's okay. Fat is delicious and it makes you feel full. As we've discussed, you need to restrict your carbohydrates to around 30 total grams per day, and you need to have between 1.2 to 2.0 grams of protein per kilogram of lean body mass per day. So, the rest needs to come from fat.

Unlike with carbohydrate and protein, there is no top number of grams you want to include in your diet. You just fill in the rest of your calories with fat. That means you put butter or oil on your vegetables. You don't bother looking for the leanest meats you can find. You use full fat everything. You will eat as many eggs as you desire. You will probably put cheese on everything and heavy whipping cream in your coffee in the morning. Unless eggs or dairy irritate you—then more oil and fatty meats.

Here are a couple of tips about fats:

1. Eat until you are satisfied. Don't add a ton of extra fat just to make sure you "hit your macros." The thing that triggers ketosis is carbohydrate restriction, not fat consumption. Just use the fat to fill in your calories and make your food delicious. You will likely find that you don't need to eat as much as you did when not eating as much fat. Fat naturally makes you feel satisfied.

2. Get your fat as naturally as possible. Fatty meats (especially fish), full-fat dairy, avocados and nuts, and minimally processed oils like extra virgin olive oil and cold pressed coconut oil are good sources. Avoid vegetable and seed oils as much as you can.

If this is your first encounter with a ketogenic diet, it is going to take some getting used to. We have been told for over 40 years that fat will kill you if you eat it. Eating a diet that is mostly fat is going to feel strange and counterintuitive. Even though your food will be delicious and you'll feel amazing, you will still likely have thoughts about how eating that much fat is going to clog your arteries and explode your heart.

To the contrary, people eating a ketogenic diet have usually shown improvements in almost every marker of cardiovascular health. Not to mention the weight loss! Carrying excess body fat is associated with a whole host of health issues. The ketogenic diet has been shown again and again to be a very effective tool for weight loss, and therefore, risk reduction. So if you get that voice in your head when you're eating your rich, delicious meals, just trust in the science, give it a month minimum, and see how you feel. Even if my mountain of scientific studies are wrong, you're not going to explode your heart in a month.

Balancing Electrolytes

Your kidneys very tightly regulate how much sodium, magnesium, and potassium leave your body in urine. During ketosis, you will lose more sodium, magnesium, and potassium through urine. It is important to replenish these minerals in adequate amounts to avoid unpleasant symptoms. Lower-than-optimal sodium levels can manifest as headache, dizziness, low energy, and something called orthostatic hypotension, which is a quick drop in blood pressure upon standing. If you've ever felt momentarily light-headed right after standing up, you've experienced orthostatic hypotension. Disrupted magnesium levels are thought to be associated with muscle cramps or twitching. Potassium regulation in the body is closely tied to sodium regulation and it is thought that "potassium follows sodium," meaning that as the concentration of sodium decreases, the body will also attempt to decrease the concentration of potassium.

To make sure your body has enough of these essential minerals and to avoid any unpleasant symptoms of your keto transition, follow these recommendations:

1. Salt your food. This is a big part of making sure you get enough sodium. When cooking, season to flavor and if you didn't cook it, add some salt at the table. Just salt to your liking, though—I'm not recommending that you pickle your tongue by going crazy with the saltshaker.

2. Drink some salt. That's an odd statement, I know. You likely need between 4 to 5 grams of sodium per day and will likely be getting 2 to 3 grams per day in your foods. If you add half a teaspoon of table salt to a glass of water a couple of times per day, you'll be getting an additional 2 to 2.5 grams of sodium. Alternately, you can drink a cup of broth, which, depending on the brand, will contain about a gram of sodium per 8 ounces. If you participate in something that makes you sweat a lot, like a hard workout or outdoor activity, you likely need even more sodium to make up for that which will be lost in sweat.

3. If you get adequate sodium and eat enough potassium-rich foods like avocados, leafy greens, broccoli, and brussels sprouts, you should not need to think about potassium supplementation.

4. Supplement magnesium. It can be difficult to get enough magnesium through diet alone. It will help you to make sure you are eating a variety of nuts, seeds, and leafy vegetables but it won't guarantee you are getting enough. If you experience muscle cramps or twitching, it is a good idea to supplement this mineral to ensure your needs are met. I recommend starting at 400 mg per day and dosing up or down from there depending on your reaction. A word of caution about magnesium supplementation: Too much can cause diarrhea. Giving patients a drink of magnesium oxide suspension is actually a standard part of constipation protocols in hospitals and long-term care facilities. To avoid disaster pants if you find that you need higher doses of magnesium supplementation, either take it as a few smaller doses throughout the day with food, or use a brand called Slo-mag that slowly releases the magnesium throughout the day.

Limit Sweeteners

I think you need to limit the use of artificial and natural sweeteners for two reasons. By artificial sweeteners, I mean the ones you typically find in "diet" processed foods: saccharin, acesulfame K, aspartame, neotame, and sucralose. I also mean sugar alcohols like sorbitol, mannitol, xylitol, and erythritol, and natural sweeteners like stevia and allulose.

There is evidence that while artificial sweeteners do not provide calories to the body, they still may induce an insulin response and they likely make you less tolerant of glucose by messing with your microbiome. If your glucose tolerance is impaired, in this context, it means you will have a lower daily carbohydrate budget.

Looking at the evidence for the sugar alcohols and the natural sweeteners is a little brighter. Sugar alcohols can be split into two categories: erythritol and everything else. Erythritol, which is not quite as sweet as regular sugar, is commercially produced and sold both in products and as a standalone sweetener. It has been shown to have either no effect or a positive effect on post-meal glucose and insulin levels, and unlike the other sugar alcohols, it does not cause uncomfortable gas and bloating.

The only notable downside to erythritol is that for some people, it produces a strange cold sensation on the tongue. That's not weird if the thing being sweetened is chewing gum or toothpaste, but it takes some getting used to for chocolate or peanut butter flavored desserts.

The rest of the sugar alcohols are pretty good from a metabolic standpoint as well. They are all metabolized to some degree and will subsequently provide some energy, but they all have relatively small effects (if any) on blood glucose levels. However, these types of sweeteners can have very unpleasant gastrointestinal side effects like bloating, diarrhea, and nausea.

The natural sugar alternatives that I've seen so far are stevia and allulose. Though I am using the word natural, note that both are obtained through industrial chemical processes, if you care about that sort of thing. Stevia is extracted from a leaf using a multi-step chemical process involving heat and some sort of solvent. Allulose is found in some whole foods like figs and jackfruit, but the allulose found in products is produced by enzymatically treating corn fructose. Both of them appear to be safe and have little to no effect on blood sugar or insulin response. Interestingly, allulose may increase fat burning after ingestion. Though it has not been studied all that well, I have heard reports of allulose causing gas and bloating similar to some of the sugar alcohols. Stevia appears to be fine.

Now for my opinion: Limit all of them. One of the points of a ketogenic diet and a carbohydrate restriction is to break your addiction to sweet foods and change your palate such that you don't need everything to be sweet. I'm not saying you can never have sweet things again and that you should not ever use these alternative sweeteners; I'm just advocating for being reasonable about it. Desserts should be relegated to a once-in-a-while sort of thing.

If you intend to make this a lifestyle change and plan to have long-term success, you have to do more than change the source of the sweetness you are craving. You have to take steps to change your expectations so that you are not craving sweetness all the time. It is much easier to abstain from carbohydrates when you are not constantly desirous of dessert. Trust me.

Alcohol in Moderation

My understanding of the available evidence is that there is no amount of alcohol that is beneficial to overall health. However, I live in the real world with you, and I know that not every choice we make is about health. You can absolutely drink while on a ketogenic diet, but do so with caution. Adhere to the same precautions you would use with alcohol under normal circumstances: don't drink and drive, be intentional about your drinking, understand that alcohol alters your decision-making abilities, be aware of the signs of alcohol poisoning, and monitor it as a potential addiction risk.

Alcohol warning out of the way, here's what you need to consider about drinking while in ketosis: Many alcoholic beverages contain carbohydrates and will need to be counted in your daily carbohydrate budget.

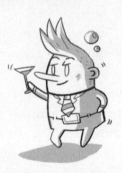

Beer. All beers contain some amount of carbohydrate and many have so many that you can't really even have one. Typically speaking, the more flavorful the beer, the more carbohydrates it contains. The only beers I have been able to include in my daily carbohydrate budget have been "light" style beers, and then typically only one or two. As with everything, just investigate until you can find a solid answer about how many carbohydrates the beer you want contains. Unlike food products, nutrition labels are not mandatory on alcohol products, so this is not always an easy task. Usually, with a little digging, the answer can be found online.

Wine. Wines are much more consistent with their carbohydrate content than beers. In general, red wines have 4 to 5 grams of carbohydrate per 4 ounces. White wines vary considerably more. I have had a much harder time finding solid information on individual wines than I have for beers, though. So if you're a wine lover, weigh the pros and cons and pay special attention to how you feel after having some wine while in ketosis.

Spirits. Most spirits will not contain any carbohydrate. This holds true across colors. Whiskey is zero carb. Vodka is zero carb. All the traditional spirits are free of carbohydrate because they have such high alcohol content. So Scotch, bourbon, rye, other whiskeys, gin, tequila, and vodka all are free from carbohydrate. You get into trouble with dessert liquors and flavored spirits.

My experience, and one I have often heard repeated, is that alcohol tolerance is diminished while eating a ketogenic diet. That may be because the kidneys are already working to clear ketone bodies from the blood, or it may be because we were not staying well enough hydrated prior to drinking the alcohol. In any case, go slow until you learn how you will react to alcohol while in ketosis.

You should now have all you need to get started on the cyclical ketogenic diet. To make it easier, I've included a 7-day meal plan on page 69.

Is this Allowed?
Adjust Your Perspective

A question I hear *all the time* from people following a ketogenic diet is, "Is this allowed?"

I think you should consider this a banned thought. It frames your food choices in terms of some rules that are outside your control. While there are factors you can't control, like how your body's metabolic framework reacts to the amount and quality of food you give it, the choice of what to put in your body is still absolutely within your control. Everything is "allowed," it just has different consequences that you will have to accept.

Instead of asking yourself if something is allowed, ask if including it in your diet will move you closer to your goals or further away. Ask yourself how your body's machinery is going to react to this input and if you are at peace with those outcomes. I understand that this is just a semantic shift, but I think it is important to recognize that you are in control of the choices you make, and understanding the consequences of those choices is the first step.

Stage 2: Weight Loss and Carb Breaks

After you've become fat adapted—at least 30 days of strict ketosis—you are ready to move onto the next stage of the cyclical ketogenic diet. The purpose of this stage is maintaining carbohydrate restriction and ketosis for as long as you need to achieve your weight-loss goals. I believe the key to being able to maintain the restrictive nature of the ketogenic diet is allowing yourself a little bit of latitude every so often. I'm calling these allowances "carb breaks," meaning a break from extreme carbohydrate restriction.

Exactly how much of a carb break you take and how often you take them is entirely up to you. To my knowledge, there is no proven advantage to cycling in and out of ketosis on a fairly regular basis. However, I am recommending that you allow yourself more carbohydrates every so often because I think it will make it easier for you to stick with the extreme carbohydrate restriction required for ketosis.

I recommend that you stick to the overall principles I've outlined regarding what you should eat during these carb breaks. They should not be junk food binges. You should think of these breaks as an opportunity to have some starchier vegetables, some fruit, or some rice.

Let's talk metabolism again to make sure you understand why I'm recommending that you keep it reasonable. It is estimated that a healthy liver can store upwards of 100 to 120 grams of glycogen. I tell you this because I want you to understand that if you go nuts and eat a whole giant mess of carbohydrates on one of your carb break days, your liver will gobble up as much of that glucose as it can and stuff it into storage. Then, it has all that stored sugar to run through before you get back into ketosis. So keep in mind that the badder your break, the longer it will take you to get back on track.

If you go off the rails entirely and have enough of a carb break to totally replenish your glycogen stores, consider having carb breaks less frequently—maybe once every 2 or 3 weeks. If you are keeping it reasonable, then maybe you can tolerate once a week. Of course, the most important thing is to pay attention to how you feel and base your carb-break practice around what you feel works best in your life.

Another reason that you don't want to go on a low-quality carbohydrate binge, especially for your first carb break after the 30 days of strict ketosis, is a metabolic quirk known as physiological insulin resistance. Physiological insulin resistance is the term for when muscle cells become resistant to the action of insulin in the context of a low-carbohydrate diet, leading to higher-than-normal blood sugar levels. It is a perfectly normal and healthy physiological response to fat adaptation. It means your muscle cells have actually come to prefer fat as fuel. However, this could be a problem during a carb break because your muscles will be less interested in using glucose and your body will choose to store that glucose as fat more quickly than it otherwise would. So heads up.

This pattern does not need to be static. It is totally fine to have a carb break once a week for 3 weeks in a row and then go a month without one. Since you've trained your body to use fats efficiently, it can switch between fuel sources much more easily and quickly. I'm basing that assertion on personal experience and understanding of metabolism. I don't know if that particular aspect of ketosis has been studied. Let's hear from Dr. Wood and the experienced team at Nourish Balance Thrive about this topic:

> *A person with a healthy metabolism should be able*
> *to switch between fuels without any significantly*
> *noticeable effects in terms of how they feel. To really*

benefit from carbohydrate cycling, though, a person
should have achieved some metabolic health first. This
could come from an initial period of carbohydrate
restriction, or making sure that their environment
has been optimized. For instance, we often restrict
carbohydrates because we have poor metabolic health,
but that poor metabolic health is because of non-dietary
causes (job/family life, poor circadian rhythm, chronic
infections, etc.), and the diet is just symptom control.
Once metabolic health has been established, adding
back small portions of carbohydrates can work well.
But slowly increase over a few weeks—don't just eat a
whole pizza in the name of carb cycling!

The flexibility afforded by our metabolic machinery allows for the life-changing benefits of ketosis while still being able to enjoy all aspects of special occasions with your friends and family. Have yourself a treat if you really need one, and live your life.

I do not recommend counting calories for the same reasons outlined regarding the accuracy of nutrient information on labels (page 51). Additionally, I regard it to be a crutch that will not be effective for long-term success. It is incredibly tedious and could be too inaccurate to be effective if your margins are thin. Weight management has to do with so much more than calories in vs. calories out that tracking your caloric intake vs. energy expenditure is not a good use of your time. Instead, pay attention to your body, your hunger and satiety cues, and try to implement as many of the lifestyle factors outlined in Chapter 6 as you can.

If you feel like you *must* track calories, then of course you should. I would recommend that you do so with an end date in mind, though. If you want to track calories in the beginning of your weight-loss journey because you have a difficult time judging how many calories you need in a day to feel satisfied, then by all means, track your calories. But pay attention to how you feel at certain calorie levels and how your body is responding. The eventual goal is to be able to eat real food in an intuitive way without losing control of your body composition. I understand that some people need metrics that are somewhat objective. That's fine. Just regard it as a transitional practice and not one that you will be employing for the rest of your life.

If you read that and thought, "How the heck do I pay attention to my hunger and satiety cues?" don't worry. Listening to our bodies is not something that many of us are accustomed to. It may take some time before you really get acclimated to the practice of intuitive eating. There are a couple of things you can do to help make the process easier. First of all, slow down. The commonly repeated wisdom is that it takes about 20 minutes for your brain to get the message that your stomach is full. Of course, it is more variable and complicated than that. How long it takes to feel full will depend on a whole bunch of complicated factors that we don't really need to talk about. However, the idea is still sound. There is some amount of lag time between when your stomach is full and when you feel full. Slowing down your meal times will give you a better chance of catching that message before you overdo it.

Continue the practice of ketosis-carb break-ketosis for as long as you need until you're happy with your body composition. After that point, move on to phase 2 of the cyclical ketogenic diet—maintenance, wellness, and longevity.

Phase 1 Sample Meal Plan

DAY 1

Breakfast
· 2 eggs, pan fried with butter

· 4 slices bacon

· 12 ounces coffee with 2 tablespoons heavy whipping cream

650 calories | 54g fat | 39g protein | 2g carbohydrate | 0g fiber | 2g net carbohydrate

Lunch
· Flank Steak and Blue Cheese Salad (page 150)

· 8 ounces water

660 calories | 56g fat | 33g protein | 12g carbohydrate | 9g fiber | 3g net carbohydrate

Dinner
· 1 serving Fontina and Sundried Tomato Stuffed Chicken Breast (page 147)

· 1 serving Herbed Mashed Cauliflower with 1 tablespoon of butter (page 170)

· 8 ounces water

642 calories | 47g fat | 39g protein | 16g carbohydrate | 5g fiber | 11g net carbohydrate

Nutrition Facts Totals for Day 1: *1,952 calories | 157g fat | 111g protein | 30g carbohydrate | 14g fiber | 16g net carbohydrate*

DAY 2

Breakfast
· 1 serving Raspberry Fontina Hotcakes (page 143)

· 12 ounces coffee with 2 tablespoons heavy whipping cream

610 calories | 54g fat | 24g protein | 5g carbohydrate | 1g fiber | 4g net carbohydrate

Lunch
- 1 slice Wonder (fully Like White) Bread (page 121), toasted with 2 tablespoons butter
- 2 ounces Brie cheese
- 8 ounces water

640 calories | 64g fat | 15g protein | 4g carbohydrate | 2g fiber | 2g net carbohydrate

Dinner
- 1 serving Ginger Bourbon Glazed Salmon (page 152)
- 1 serving Sage-Roasted Broccoli (page 173)
- 2 ounces bourbon
- 8 ounces water

585 calories | 24g fat | 25g protein | 19g carbohydrate | 5g fiber | 14g net carbohydrate

Nutrition Facts Totals for Day 2: *1,835 calories | 142g fat | 64g protein | 28g carbohydrate | 8g fiber | 20g net carbohydrate*

DAY 3

Breakfast
- Parmlette (page 142)
- 12 ounces coffee with 2 tablespoons heavy whipping cream

580 calories | 41g fat | 30g protein | 10g carbohydrate | 6g fiber | 4g net carbohydrate

Lunch
- 1 serving Crispy Spiced Chicken Tenders (page 148)
- Side salad with lettuce, olives, celery, and olive oil
- 8 ounces unsweetened tea

659 calories | 59g fat | 26g protein | 10g carbohydrate | 9g fiber | 1g net carbohydrate

Dinner
- 1 (8 ounce) sirloin steak, cooked in Cilantro Lime Chili Butter (page 189)

- 1 serving Roasted Cabbage (page 174)
- 1 serving Lemon Zest Yogurt Cake (page 181)
- 8 ounces water

  661 calories | 45g fat | 54g protein | 8g carbohydrate | 5g fiber | 3g net carbohydrate

Nutrition Facts Totals for Day 3: *1,900 calories | 145g fat | 110g protein | 28g carbohydrate | 20g fiber | 8g net carbohydrate*

DAY 4

Breakfast
- 3-egg omelet
  » 1 ounce cheddar cheese
  » 1 tablespoon butter
  » 2 slices bacon, crumbled
  » 1 tablespoon sour cream
- 12 ounces coffee with 2 tablespoons heavy whipping cream

  689 calories | 58g fat | 37g protein | 2g carbohydrate | 0g fiber | 2g net carbohydrate

Lunch
- 1 serving Tuna Salad Zucchini Boats (page 151)
- ½ avocado
- 8 ounces green tea with 1 tablespoon coconut oil

  582 calories | 46g fat | 19g protein | 10g carbohydrate | 6g fiber | 4g net carbohydrate

Dinner
- 1 serving Peanut Chicken Kabobs (page 155)
- ½ cup riced cauliflower
- 2 tablespoons butter

  660 calories | 42g fat | 53g protein | 18g carbohydrate | 7g fiber | 11g net carbohydrate

Nutrition Facts Totals for Day 4: *1,931 calories | 146g fat | 109g protein | 30g carbohydrate | 13g fiber | 17g net carbohydrate*

DAY 5

Breakfast
- 1 serving Perfect Keto Muffins (page 126)
- 1 tablespoon butter
- 1 ounce macadamia nuts
- 12 ounces coffee with 2 tablespoons heavy whipping cream

579 calories | 56g fat | 8g protein | 10g carbohydrate | 4g fiber | 6g net carbohydrate

Lunch
- salad with lettuce, olives, celery, chicken, goat cheese, and Magic Olive Oil and Vinegar Dressing (page 190)
- 8 ounces Electroaide (page 186)

600 calories | 47g fat | 39g protein | 5g carbohydrate | 5g fiber | 0g net carbohydrate

Dinner
- 1 (4 ounce) pork chop
- 1 zucchini, spiralized
- 2 tablespoons extra virgin olive oil
- 1 serving Bolognese sauce (page 192)
- 2 tablespoons shredded Parmigiano-Reggiano cheese
- 8 ounces water

725 calories | 56g fat | 45g protein | 11g carbohydrate | 3g fiber | 8g net carbohydrate

Nutrition Facts Totals for Day 5: *1,904 calories | 159g fat | 92g protein | 26g carbohydrate | 12g fiber | 14g net carbohydrate*

DAY 6

Breakfast
- 1 serving Everything Bagel (Flavored) Biscuits (page 119)
- 2 ounces cream cheese
- 2 ounces smoked salmon
- 12 ounces coffee

500 calories | 40g fat | 19g protein | 7g carbohydrate | 2g fiber | 5g net carbohydrate

Lunch
- snack plate
  » 1 serving Baked Brie (page 138)
  » 3 mini bell peppers stuffed with Crème Fraîche (page 135)
  » 2 ounces pancetta
  » 2 ounces capicola
  » 1 ounce almonds
- 8 ounces water

691 calories | 55g fat | 35g protein | 15g carbohydrate | 7g fiber | 8g net carbohydrate

Dinner
- 1 serving Caprese Hasselback Chicken (page 146)
- 1 serving Sesame Zucchini Rounds (page 172)
- 8 ounces water
- 2 servings Strawberry Cream Gummies (page 184)

566 calories | 46g fat | 34g protein | 6g carbohydrate | 2g fiber | 4g net carbohydrate

Nutrition Facts Totals for Day 6: *1,757 calories | 141g fat | 88g protein | 28g carbohydrate | 11g fiber | 17g net carbohydrate*

DAY 7

Breakfast · 1 serving Raspberry Muffin Egg and Cheese
Sandwich (page 144)

· 12 ounces coffee with 2 tablespoons heavy
whipping cream

*564 calories | 51g fat | 20g protein | 8g carbohydrate |
3g fiber | 5g net carbohydrate*

Lunch · 1 serving Buffalo Chicken Stuffed Poblano
Peppers (page 154)

· 2 servings Garlic and Onion Parmesan Crisps

*530 calories | 38g fat | 33g protein | 13g carbohydrate |
4g fiber | 9g net carbohydrate*

Dinner · ribeye steak, cooked in butter

· 1 serving Turnips Au Gratin (page 175)

· 8 ounces water

*925 calories | 91g fat | 61g protein | 7g carbohydrate |
2g fiber | 5g net carbohydrate*

Nutrition Facts Totals for Day 7: *2,019 calories | 180g fat | 114g protein
| 28g carbohydrate | 9g fiber | 19g net carbohydrate*

I understand I told you to follow a strict ketogenic diet for at
least 30 days but didn't give you a whole 30 days of recipes. Fret
not! Chapter 7 is a good place to start, and the internet is just
stuffed to the gills with low-carb recipes. But don't take them
at face value. Make sure they are actually low carb enough to
fit into your budget. I've seen a lot of websites claiming to have
recipes appropriate for a ketogenic diet that are, well, not. Just
be cautious and do due diligence.

Main Takeaways

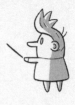

1. Restrict your carbohydrate intake to 20 to 30 grams per day for no less than 30 days. This allows you to become fat adapted and makes it easier to jump in and out of ketosis.

2. After you're fat adapted, allow yourself carb breaks as often as you feel like you need to while still making progress toward your goals. The frequency of breaks will depend on how many carbohydrates you eat during a carb break.

3. Continue cycling until you meet your weight loss or body composition goals.

Chapter Five

The Cyclical Ketogenic Diet Phase 2:
Maintenance and Wellness

By the time you are ready to approach this phase, you will have been following a cyclical ketogenic diet for at least 30 days, but likely longer. Your body should be very good at using both fat and glucose for fuel at this point. This phase of the cyclical ketogenic diet involves making that metabolic switch on a fairly regular basis. It is intended to be a lifestyle and lifelong change. In this chapter, I will help you understand the principles of healthy low-carb eating by outlining some overarching heuristics that you can use to make sure you are effortlessly eating well on an ongoing basis.

Your body composition should be at or pretty close to where you would like it to be by the time you transition into this phase. Now, your priority will be maintaining a healthy weight, nourishing your body appropriately, and promoting overall wellness.

Moving forward, you will not necessarily be intentionally restricting grams of carbohydrate, but your intake of carbohydrates will be low by virtue of how your diet is structured. You will still be eating a moderate amount of high-quality protein, a lot of healthy fats, and filling the rest in with high-fiber, low-carbohydrate fruits and vegetables. The difference here is that you will include more fruits and a wider variety of vegetables. Most grains and all refined sugars will still be excluded unless you choose to include them on an irregular basis as a treat. In addition to food composition, meal timing is important for phase 2 of the cyclical ketogenic diet, and you'll be flirting with some intermittent fasting.

Evaluating Foods

This phase of the cyclical ketogenic diet is much more liberal and will cycle you into ketosis on a pretty regular, but less formulaic, basis. I don't want you to worry about grams of anything but instead focus on two main concepts: nutrient density, and the idea that everything you put in your body will either be a nourishing benefit or an antagonistic detriment to your overall health and wellness goals. When combined, these two concepts are very powerful and can help you build a nourishing, healthful, and intuitive eating style. I hope for you to change the way that you think of food in a general sense as well as a specific sense. I want the choices you are making about food to become automatic so that eventually, making good and healthful choices are not taxing and don't require any of your finite willpower day in and day out.

Nutrient density is basically a way to evaluate food based on how much nutrition it will provide. By nutrition, I mean calories, essential amino acids, essential fatty acids, fiber, vitamins, and minerals. The concept of nutrient density can be applied in broad strokes. You are always trying to get the best nutritional bang for your caloric buck, and you are almost always going to be able to do that by sticking with minimally processed whole foods. It doesn't take much thought to know that broccoli is going to be more nutritionally dense than a brownie.

The second guideline, evaluate everything in terms of nourishment vs. antagonism, is a little less intuitive than nutrient density, but I'm going to give you some pointers for some things to look out for in foods that may lead to antagonism over nourishment.

What to Eat

Much like phase 1 of the cyclical ketogenic diet, you want to emphasize whole foods whenever you can, include high-quality fats and protein sources, eat lots of vegetables, and avoid concentrated sources of carbohydrates like breads, pastas, and sugary desserts. Phase 2 differs in that you will be including a wider variety of vegetables, including starchy vegetables, and having more fruit.

So let's say your meal would have been a 3- to 4-ounce portion of steak or chicken seared in butter, some sautéed spinach with garlic and olive oil, and an almond flour-based biscuit during phase 1. Now, instead of spinach, you could include some sweet potato mash (no brown sugar), some rice, or a medium ear of corn. You're still aiming to get adequate protein to maintain your tissue and build muscle. You still want to use fat to flavor your foods and make you feel satisfied. You're just limiting carbohydrate a bit less now. The same general principles apply with sweets and sweeteners that I outlined in phase 1 (page 60).

As I said above, I don't want you to have to think about grams, but depending on how much you eat in a day, you'll likely be eating between 50 to 100 grams of carbohydrates daily in this phase.

Many health pundits have repeated the maxim "If it has a label, don't eat it." While that general principle is good, I think we all understand that is a bit unrealistic. I'd like to modify that idea a bit: If it has a label, has more than five ingredients, and you can't pronounce one or more of those ingredients, *then* you should definitely skip it. Aside from that, you're just going to have to use your judgment when incorporating foods with labels.

Your higher carbohydrate limit opens up a lot of possibilities for food choices. You can now enjoy a seasonally appropriate fruit as a dessert or ingredient in a meal. Beans and rice are back on the menu. Lentils are a go. Remember, this is not an invitation to go back to the eating habits you had before starting the cyclical ketogenic diet.

As a very general rule, you should shop the periphery of the store and stick to whole foods you will have to cook. By "the periphery," I do actually mean the edges of the store. This tends to be where the produce, dairy, meats, and seafood are sold. Of course, it is more complicated than that and there are some things you need to try to avoid in those sections. Let's talk about what to avoid.

The Abstinence Violation Effect

This portion of the diet has fewer hard rules, which can be dangerous for some people. I personally do better if I have harder restrictions, and it has taken me several years of effort to make avoidance of processed foods and added sugars my default setting.

There is a nasty psychological trick known as the abstinence violation effect (AVE) I want you to watch out for. Basically, AVE is when a person has decided to abstain from a substance (like sugar) or behavior (like skipping your workout) but they use that substance or participate in that behavior. The breaking of the abstinence (eating a cupcake) is not the nasty psychological trick; the trick happens afterward. Some people, myself included, struggle with deciding that, since they've already "messed up," they may as well give up. That's what happens when one bad bite becomes one bad meal, then a day of bad meals, then a week. Before you know it, you've abandoned your resolve altogether and may have to start all over again.

While this thought process is very common, it does not have to be inevitable. Remember that every single bite you take is a choice and it does not have to influence the next bite you take. If you slip up and eat something you should not, don't allow it to derail you for any longer than that single decision. If you think of every choice as an opportunity to either advance you closer to your goals or take you farther from them, it becomes easier to recover from missteps.

What to Avoid

While you don't need to count grams and fret over macronutrient composition, there are still some food items you would be better off to avoid. There are some obvious ones, like highly processed food-like items (think Coke and Pop-Tarts), but there are a few others that are worth consideration. Grains, inflammatory oils, and factory-farmed meat are all things you would likely be better off avoiding. Of course, you may be able to tolerate any of these just fine, but you should be aware of the potential pros and cons of including them in your diet.

Grains

Grains, particularly gluten-containing grains, can have suboptimal effects on your diet. That is to say, some people are truly allergic to them, others are irritated by them, and still others do not notice any ill effects of consumption. People who are allergic to the protein complex gluten have a condition called celiac disease, and their reaction to gluten is so profound that it usually prompts them to seek medical attention. Celiac disease can manifest as a wide variety of symptoms ranging from diarrhea to numbness in the extremities. The only treatment is total, lifelong avoidance of gluten.

Many others have reported less severe, but still quite irritating, symptoms following the ingestion of gluten. The symptoms reported tend to be somewhat nebulous like upset stomach, generalized fatigue, or brain fog. Though there is no scientific consensus on this topic, some medical practitioners recognize this as a condition known as gluten intolerance or non-celiac gluten sensitivity. There is no validated test for gluten intolerance, but symptoms generally improve when gluten is eliminated from the diet.

Finally, there are those that will not have any noticeable symptoms from eating gluten. Unfortunately, I believe that harm is still being done. The reason that I think gluten-containing grains are worth avoiding for just about everyone has to do with the small intestine, its immune function, and a protein called zonulin. Let's take a detour into the physiology of the gut for a moment.

In addition to being the primary site of nutrient absorption, your small intestine also serves as one of the front lines of your immune system. There are complex systems in place that screen the material passing through your small intestine, searching for the vital nutrition your body needs but also for pathogens and irritants that can harm you. If your system is working optimally, your intestinal wall will only allow the nutrients to pass through into your bloodstream.

One of the main features of this biological security system is the wall of the gut. The cells in your gut wall are held together very tightly by thread-like proteins that stitch them together. They are stitched so tightly that nothing can pass

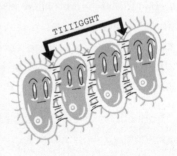

through the space in between cells. These connections are called "tight junctions," and in healthy people, they keep out the larger molecules from your food that could be problematic, such as viruses, bacteria, and incompletely digested proteins.

Zonulin is a protein in your body that signals for the threads holding these tight junctions to relax and increase the space between your gut wall cells. So far, the scientific community has only identified two things that will prompt the release of zonulin and subsequent relaxation of the tight junctions of the gut wall: certain bacteria and gluten. So the protein compound gluten, found in many grains, induces the security system in your gut to relax and possibly allow viruses, bacteria, and partially digested proteins to directly enter your bloodstream. Viruses and bacteria are obviously an issue because they can directly cause illness. Large, partially digested proteins are a problem, too. Because these proteins have not been broken down into the small form that your body is used to seeing, your immune system may treat these proteins as a threat.

If the immune system is chronically activated because you are chronically eating gluten, which is chronically opening your gut wall, you run the risk of several complications. First, chronic immune response will inevitably do some collateral damage to your own cells. This is part of what is referred to as inflammation, which is undesirable when it occurs chronically. Many diseases are associated with chronic inflammation either as part of the disease process or potentially as part of the cause. There are some models of heart disease that point to chronic, low-level inflammation as the driving force behind atherosclerosis and eventual cardiac events like heart attack and stroke. So, clearly chronic inflammation is something you want to avoid.

Gluten promotes this relaxation of intestinal tight junctions in all people, not just those with a gluten allergy or intolerance. However, it appears that in individuals that do not have celiac disease or gluten intolerance, the degree of increased intestinal permeability is not as severe and does not last as long. So, your gut will only leak toxins into your bloodstream for a little while after you eat gluten.

Obviously, not everyone that eats gluten will get a viral or bacterial infection, or develop an autoimmune disease. Billions of people have been eating gluten for generations without an obvious increase in these issues. Some health advocates argue that the type of grains (and gluten) we have in our food supply are somehow fundamentally different from what humans evolved eating. Others claim that our production methods have changed such that the gluten is more complete when we eat it than it would have been in the past. Still others argue that our relative load of gluten has increased due to the amount of bready products we eat on a daily basis. As with many things, I suspect the truth may be a combination of these factors.

In my opinion, gluten-containing grains are a long shot from being necessary in your diet, and there is the possibility that they are causing you some amount of harm—or, at least increasing the possibility of harm from other sources. They are also, obviously, mostly carbohydrate, which you are trying to limit in your diet. I know they are delicious, convenient, and ubiquitous, but are they worth the risk?

Industrial Oils

While you definitely do not need to fear fats and you still want to use fat as your caloric and satiety filler during this phase of the cyclical ketogenic diet, not all fats are created equal. And even if they were, the fats I'm going to recommend you avoid don't look anything like they did when they were created by the time you would be eating them. The oils I'm referring to are the highly processed seed oils found in a disturbing amount of our food supply. That would include canola or rapeseed oil, safflower oil, corn oil, soy oil, mixtures sold as "vegetable oil," and any oil that has been partially hydrogenated.

The biggest sources of these types of oils are processed and commercially fried foods that you should be avoiding anyway. So that should reduce your consumption of them quite a lot. Still, you are going to need oils occasionally for cooking. Here are some reasons to avoid industrial seed oils when cooking.

1. They are flavorless. Really, when you're cooking, you want every ingredient to bring something to the table from a nutrition and a flavor perspective. These oils are not devoid of nutrition, but they are pretty much devoid of flavor. That should be reason enough to choose something else.

2. They are unstable. All oils are sensitive to a process called oxidation in which they become less chemically stable and more dangerous once they get into your body. For this reason, you want any oil you choose to include in your diet to be as stable as possible. Oxidation of oils is caused by a variety of factors including age, light exposure, chemical exposure, heat, and metal content. Yeah, you read that correctly—the oils we eat have some metal in them. Anyway, industrially processed oils tend to be very sensitive to the process of oxidation.

3. The ratio of fats in your diet matters. Though the science community disagrees somewhat about whether omega-6 fats (the primary fatty acids found in industrial oils) are pro-inflammatory or anti-inflammatory, there is relative agreement that the ratio of omega-6 to omega-3 fatty acids in the diet appears to matter in terms of inflammation and the progression of obesity, cardiovascular disease, cancer, autoimmune diseases, and dementia. It is thought that before the introduction of processed seed oils and the industrial food supply, the ratio of omega-6 to omega-3 in our diets ranged from 1:1 to 4:1. It is now in the range of 15:1 to 25:1. If your diet is primarily whole foods and you do not use industrial oils in your own cooking, you should have a much better ratio. Maybe not 1:1 as our ancestors did, but closer.

Partially hydrogenated oils get their own special mention: avoid them altogether. They have no place in your diet. Hydrogenation is the process of taking an unsaturated fatty acid and adding hydrogen atoms to its carbon chain. This is done to give the fat more favorable properties (from an industrial food production perspective), like shelf stability and a moist mouthfeel. A chemical side effect of this process is a change to the structure of the fatty acid chain, which is pretty bad in the human body. These altered fatty acids are known as trans fats. Artificially produced trans fats are strongly associated with an increased risk of cardiovascular disease. Plus, you will only find them in gross stuff you should be avoiding, like those prepackaged muffins found at gas stations with several-year-long shelf lives.

Oh, and a quick note about nutrition label shenanigans: If you do choose to eat something like that and you check the label because you still want to avoid trans fat, be careful. If "partially hydrogenated" anything is one of the ingredients, it contains trans fats no matter what the nutrition label says. The FDA allows for anything containing less than .05 grams trans fat *per serving* to list the trans fat as zero.

Factory-Farmed Meat

If you care about animal welfare or environmental sustainability, your health, or the health of your family (surely you care about at least one of those things), you want to avoid meat that comes from the industrial food supply as much as is feasible.

Without getting into any very nasty details, I will say that the conditions factory-farmed animals are subjected to is flat-out horrific. Each year, billions of animals are raised and slaughtered in industrial farms under conditions that most of us would find unacceptable. Overcrowding, poor air and light quality, filth that leads to illness, inappropriate feed, neglect, and abuse are common in this type of meat production system. If you are interested in learning more about the conditions of animals in our factory food supply or about some of the politics behind it, I recommend the excellent book by Jonathan Safran Foer, *Eating Animals*. It is an honest, well researched, and heartbreaking account of the writer's investigation into how his food is produced, following the birth of his first child.

From an environmental perspective, factory-farmed meat is an issue both in the communities where these farms are physically located and worldwide. Locally, they are an issue because of the volume of waste produced by such a large quantity of animals in one place. The problem is just staggering and producers have not come up with a very good solution. Currently, factory farm waste is stored in what are called "anaerobic lagoons" by the industry and "waste lagoons" by everyone else. They are huge, open-air holes filled with urine, blood, pus, and feces. When they overfill, the sludge is liquefied and sprayed over fields as fertilizer. These lagoons have been shown to leak toxins and antibiotics into the soil and groundwater. Additionally, people in the communities in which these lagoons are located tend to have higher rates of nausea, high blood pressure, and respiratory issues like asthma—and they complain that their neighborhoods smell like "death."

Volume is also an issue with factory farming on a global scale. Because of the sheer volume of meat being produced, much of the Earth's landmass is being used either for the animals themselves or to grow food for the animals. Industrial meat production is responsible for much of the deforestation that has occurred in the last few decades. When a biologically diverse ecosystem is razed and replaced with a factory lot or mono-culture grain operation, there are dire consequences in terms of carbon sequestering and biodiversity. The industrial meat system also uses an obscene amount of water and produces an obscene amount of climate change–inducing methane gas.

Most relevant to this book, however, are the health effects of factory farm-produced meat. The meat that comes out of the factory farming system is lower quality than the meat from animals that were raised and fed closer to how they would be in nature. This holds true across all categories of animal prod-uct. The meat from animals raised and killed in the industrial production system tend to have a worse fatty acid profile, lower levels of antioxidants, lower vitamin and mineral content, and (though this is subjective) less flavor.

As if the lower nutritional consequences of the industrial meat supply was not bad enough, a larger issue with this system is the overuse of antibiotics and subsequent rise of antibiotic-resistant strains of bacteria. Antibiotic-resistant bacteria are just what they sound like: pathogenic strains of bacteria that are able to withstand antibiotics. Obviously, they are bad for humans because we are running out of alternate ways to treat them and there may soon come a day when, if you get infected by one of these bacterial strains, there will be no treatment options available. The industrial meat industry is responsible for the rise of antibiotic-resistant strains of bacteria more than any other factor because they routinely use more antibiotics than any other industry. Because of the filthy conditions inside these factories, the animals get sick—a lot—so the producers give them lots of antibiotics. Some places even add the antibiotics to the animals' feed on a routine basis to attempt to prevent illness and speed growth. This leads to more opportunities for the bacteria lines to mutate and more opportunities for resistant strains to develop.

Unfortunately, all this nastiness applies to eggs and dairy, as well. In all, it is a very troubling system that you should avoid funding. However, as with all my recommendations, they are intended to be followed under optimal conditions, and I understand that life is not always optimal. Avoiding factory-farmed meat altogether is a very difficult thing to do given our food system. Most of the meat available for purchase in America comes from factory farms and it is certainly economically reinforced—in other words, it is cheaper. If you even have alternative sources for meat in your area, the cost can be much higher than just going to the grocery store. It is important that we all do what we can to incentivize sustainable and just systems for producing meat. But, it is also important to pay our monthly bills. Do the best you can.

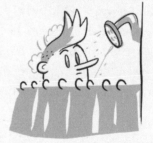

WHY ARE WE ALWAYS SAYING "FOOD IS MEDICINE" BUT FIND IT SO HARD TO ADMIT THAT SOME FOOD IS POISON??

When to Eat

There is a growing body of evidence showing the power of meal timing, or, put in a different way, the power of eating only when our bodies evolved to be eating. The act of eating does more to our bodies than simply provide them with fuel. Every time we eat, we are initiating a complex system of signals and hormones. We have a pretty good handle on the balance of insulin, the hormone that takes fuel from your bloodstream and gets it into your cells, and glucagon, the hormone that tells the stored fuel in your cells to mobilize into your bloodstream. Other aspects we don't understand as well, like how the body's circadian rhythm regulates metabolism.

Circadian rhythm is the term given to the body's natural cycle of activity and rest. This rhythm has been observed in all biological life and really bad things happen if it is severely disrupted. The most obvious example of the circadian rhythm is the sleep-wake cycle. If a person is perpetually awake when the body should be asleep and vice versa, it appears to have negative health consequences. People who work night or swing shifts often have worse health outcomes than those of us fortunate enough to be able to sleep at night and be awake during the day. There is even a medically recognized condition known as shift work syndrome, and it is associated with a greater risk of cancer, heart disease, metabolic disorder, and menstrual disruption. Though we don't fully understand it yet, it looks like eating in agreement with your natural circadian rhythm has powerful metabolic benefits.

We, as a society, have gotten into the bad habit of eating almost constantly. We eat breakfast as soon as we wake up, we have a sugar-laden latte on the way to work, we have our mid-morning work snack, then lunch, an afternoon snack, dinner, and a bedtime snack. I'm being hyperbolic but you get the point. It even became weight-loss advice to eat constantly. You all remember how we were advised to eat six meals a day to "keep your metabolism active all day," whatever that means.

In reality, what we are doing by eating all the time is keeping our insulin levels high and preventing our bodies from being able to burn fat in a meaningful way. Our bodies likely evolved to go through periods of feast *and* famine. That is likely the whole reason we store fat in the way that we do, and the reason we can thrive by living off that stored fat for such long periods.

Time-Restricted Eating and Intermittent Fasting

There are several varieties of intermittent fasting and they can all be powerful tools to help you meet your goals and take your health back. I asked an expert on fasting and the ketogenic diet, Kristen Mancinelli, to give an overview of intermittent fasting and its various forms.

Intermittent fasting is an approach to "timed eating" that lets you make the most of the body's ability to burn stored fat between meals. Unlike a typical diet, you don't have to change what you eat. Instead, you'll create eating times and fasting times, and eat only during eating times.

You see, you don't burn fat at the same rate all the time. Right after a meal, almost no stored fat is being burned. The contribution of fat to your energy needs increases steadily and peaks 18 to 24 hours after a meal. So, if you can stick it out and avoid eating for almost a day, you'll get maximum fat burning in that last 6 hours of fasting! Even shorter fasts allow you to burn more stored fat. A common practice is to fast for 16 hours and keep your eating window to 8 hours. Sixteen hours of fasting is long enough to deplete glycogen, or stored glucose, in the liver. Once glycogen is depleted, the body turns to fat for energy, and you begin to get the benefits of fasting.

It's not as hard as it sounds. For one thing, your sleep time counts toward your fasting time, so that's 8 hours right there. If you skip breakfast and stop eating after dinner you can do a 12 p.m. to 8 p.m. eating window and get the benefits of using fat for energy outside that period.

A lot of people like the daily fast of at least 16 hours and up to 24 hours. In the latter, you eat one meal a day at the same time (say, 7 p.m.) every day. Other people prefer what's called the 5:2 method where you eat normally five days a week and fast completely, or have very few calories, (e.g., 500 to 600 calories) for two days per week. Still others will fast every other day, so there is a period of normal eating alternating with a day of no eating (or eating only about 500 calories).

So your goal should be to have some meaningful amount of time between your meals. You are not necessarily looking to eat less, just less often. As you see, there are many different styles of intermittent fasting to choose from. The style that you choose is not all that important, so long as you pick one that fits with your schedule and that you enjoy. Maybe skipping breakfast is easy for you because you're always rushing out the *door anyway. Maybe you want to do one meal a day because you love sitting down with your family in the evening but don't like taking a break from your work in the middle of the day.*

An easy way to incorporate circadian timing and intermittent fasting is to allow the sun to dictate your eating window. You can eat when the sun is up and avoid eating when it is not. Obviously, the amount of daylight you experience will vary based on season and location but in general, you're looking at about 12 hours of daylight and 12 hours of night. If you just follow this simple heuristic, you will get at least 12 hours of fasting per day, which is an improvement from the current standard. As Mancinelli pointed out above, most of that fast is sleeping time anyway. If you throw in a skipped breakfast, you've easily made it to a 16 hour fast and have likely gone most of the way to depleting your glycogen stores.

Whatever you choose, I advise that your eating window close at least two hours before you plan to be asleep. There is evidence that eating, particularly a heavy caloric load, will reduce both quality and quantity of sleep.

We've talked about the way that fasting promotes fat metabolism (which is always a good thing), but evidence is mounting that there is a robust host of health benefits to intermittent fasting. There are some obvious ones, like an increase in insulin sensitivity, glucose regulation, and blood-lipid profiles, but it appears that there are a host of other benefits as well.

In addition to reducing total fat mass, researchers have found that intermittent fasting tends to change fat cells from the white type of fat cell to the brown type of fat cell. This is important because white fat cells store calories and brown fat cells burn calories. So by incorporating some fasting into your routine, you are not only directly losing weight but also protecting yourself against future weight gain.

Fasting may also protect you against some of the unpleasant aspects of aging in general. Improvements in inflammation and oxidative damage have been observed at a cellular level in people participating in some type of fasting. Importantly, these cellular protections were seen both during fasting and after breaking a fast.

There is even some evidence that intermittent fasting can improve mood and energy in otherwise healthy people. Though, as Mancinelli outlined above, there are several types of fasting protocols to choose from, and the research mentioned above used a bunch of different types. So I can't guarantee that a 12-hour fast will provide all the benefits mentioned, but I'm pretty confident saying that greater than 12 and less than 24 is the way to go for finding the sweet spot between sustainability and benefit.

Metabolic Flexibility

Another benefit of eating a whole food, lowish-carbohydrate diet and incorporating some degree of intermittent fasting is that you will develop and maintain robust metabolic flexibility. The idea of metabolic flexibility is just what you think it would be: the body's ability to easily use a variety of fuel sources and switch between

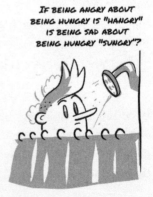

IF BEING ANGRY ABOUT BEING HUNGRY IS "HANGRY" IS BEING SAD ABOUT BEING HUNGRY "SUNGRY"?

those fuel sources seamlessly. This means you will be able to quickly and efficiently burn the carbohydrates that you eat and rely on fats when you don't eat carbohydrates (or don't eat all), without feeling any low energy or getting "hangry."

You can think of metabolic flexibility as a pretty good proxy measure for your overall metabolic health. If your body is able to use a variety of fuels easily, it is a pretty good indication that your mitochondria are in good shape. Mitochondria are the power plants of our cells and both their number and efficiency are very important for overall energy level and metabolic function.

The things that we know affect metabolic flexibility are exercise (we'll get to that in the next chapter), fat adaptation, fasting, and the inclusion of fiber, plant polyphenols, and omega-3 fatty acids in the diet. If you'll recall, all these things are a part of the cyclical ketogenic diet.

What About Ketosis?

This book is called *The Cyclical Ketogenic Diet*, yet I'm going on and on about whole foods and intermittent fasting. Don't feel tricked! We're still talking about ketosis, and you will be sliding in and out of ketosis on a regular basis if you are following the above recommendations.

As you recall, the only requisite for the body to produce and use ketones is not having enough glucose to meet the body's energy requirements. This forces the breakdown of fat and the subsequent production of ketones. Following the above principles for your meal selection, in combination with the meal timing and intermittent fasting, will lead to a natural cycle in which you are almost constantly depleting and refilling your glycogen stores. This will lead to periods in which you don't replenish quickly enough and you spend portions of the day, or possibly full days, in ketosis. It will depend on the food choices and meal timing choices you make, as well as your activity level for those days.

So even though you're not going to be obsessively tracking your carbs, calories, or anything else you will be getting much of the metabolic, epigenetic, and anti-inflammatory benefits of the ketogenic diet. All while eating sweet potatoes!

A couple of notes about this meal plan: You'll notice that breakfast each day includes only black coffee. This is the incorporation of intermittent fasting that we discussed earlier. Also notice that while these meals include more grams of carbohydrate, they still include considerably less than you would find in a typical SAD meal.

Phase 2 Sample Meal Plan

DAY 1

Breakfast · 12 ounces coffee, black

Lunch · nachos

» 2 servings Tortilla Chips (page 128)

» 1 serving Buffalo Chicken Dip (page 177)

» 1 serving Creamy Cheese Sauce (page 191)

» 2 tablespoons salsa of choice

» 1 tablespoon sour cream

» 1 tablespoon diced red onion

· 8 ounces water

955 calories | 84g fat | 38g protein | 14g carbohydrate | 5g fiber | 9g net carbohydrate

Dinner   · 1 serving Deconstructed Philly Cheese Steak (page 156)

· 1 serving Sweet Potato Buttermilk Drop Biscuits (page 124)

· 8 ounces water

· 1 serving Coconut Avocado Fiesta Pops (page 180)

920 calories | 73g fat | 33g protein | 33g carbohydrate | 15g fiber | 18g net carbohydrate

Nutrition Facts Totals for Day 1: *1875 calories | 157g fat | 71g protein | 47g carbohydrate | 20g fiber | 27g net carbohydrate*

DAY 2

Breakfast   · 12 ounces coffee, black

Lunch   · 2 servings Spinach and Cream Cheese Dumplings (page 160)

· 2 servings Ginger Beef Dumplings (page 158)

· ½ cup brown rice

· Soy sauce, to taste

· 8 ounces water

1,080 calories | 81g fat | 44g protein | 49g carbohydrate | 9g fiber | 40g net carbohydrate

Dinner   · 1 serving Beef Stew (page 162)

· 2 servings Cheddar Jalapeno "Corn" Bread (page 123)

· 8 ounces water

1,098 calories | 66g fat | 46g protein | 33g carbohydrate | 7g fiber | 26g net carbohydrate

Nutrition Facts Totals for Day 2: *2,178 calories | 147g fat | 90g protein | 82g carbohydrate | 16g fiber | 66g net carbohydrate*

DAY 3

Breakfast · 12 ounces coffee, black

Lunch · 1 serving Sausage and Rosemary Stuffed Acorn Squash (page 164)

· 1 serving Baked Okra (page 176)

· Side salad with lettuce, shredded cheddar, walnuts, onions, and bacon crumbles

· 8 ounces water

877 calories | 66g fat | 38g protein | 36g carbohydrate | 10g fiber | 26g net carbohydrate

Dinner · 1 (8 ounce) sirloin cooked with butter

· 1 medium sweet potato

· 1 tablespoon butter

· 8 ounces water

· 1 serving Cheesecake (page 182)

896 calories | 61g fat | 53g protein | 33g carbohydrate | 7g fiber | 26g net carbohydrate

Nutrition Facts Totals for Day 3: *1,773 calories | 127g fat | 91g protein | 69g carbohydrate | 17g fiber | 52g net carbohydrate*

DAY 4

Breakfast · 12 ounces coffee, black

Lunch · 1 (6 ounce) baked chicken breast

· ½ cup asparagus sautéed with olive oil

· 1 serving Butternut Squash, Sage, and Apple Soup (page 166)

· 1 serving Fat Head Bread (page 134)

· 8 ounces water

- 2 tablespoons mascarpone cheese with 5 or 6 blueberries

  810 calories | 57g fat | 43g protein | 48g carbohydrate | 10g fiber | 38g net carbohydrate

Dinner
- 1 (8-ounce) pork chop
- 2 servings Spicy Collard Greens (page 178)
- ½ cup green beans with 2 tablespoons butter
- 8 ounces water
- 1 serving Blueberry Chia Pudding (page 185)

  1,042 calories | 64g fat | 72g protein | 47g carbohydrate | 33g fiber | 14g net carbohydrate

Nutrition Facts Totals for Day 4: *1,852 calories | 121g fat | 115g protein | 95g carbohydrate | 43g fiber | 52g net carbohydrate*

DAY 5

Breakfast
- 12 ounces coffee, black

Lunch
- lettuce burger
  » 1 (½-pound) hamburger patty
  » 2 ounces cheddar cheese
  » 2 large iceberg or romaine lettuce leaves
  » 1 slice tomato
  » 1 slice onion
  » Condiments of choice (no low-quality mayonnaise!)
- Baked potato with sour cream, butter, and bacon crumbles
- 8 ounces water

  1,010 calories | 57g fat | 36g protein | 38g carbohydrate | 4g fiber | 34g net carbohydrate

Dinner	· Flank Steak and Blue Cheese Salad (page 150)
	· 8 ounces water
	· 1 serving Coconut Avocado Fiesta Pops (page 180)

831 calories | 70g fat | 34g protein | 18g carbohydrate | 15g fiber | 3g net carbohydrate

Nutrition Facts Totals for Day 5: *1,841 calories | 127g fat | 70g protein | 56g carbohydrate | 19g fiber | 37g net carbohydrate*

DAY 6

Breakfast	· 12 ounces coffee, black
Lunch	· 3 eggs, pan fried with butter
	· 4 slices bacon
	· ½ avocado
	· 1 serving Perfect Keto Muffins (page 126)

907 calories | 72g fat | 52g protein | 13g carbohydrate | 7g fiber | 6g net carbohydrate

Dinner	· 1 serving Ginger Bourbon Glazed Salmon (page 152)
	· 1 serving Sage-Roasted Broccoli (page 173)
	· 1 medium sweet potato, baked with butter and cinnamon
	· 3½ ounces red wine
	· 8 ounces water
	· 1 serving Cheesecake (page 182)

1,220 calories | 77g fat | 33g protein | 52g carbohydrate | 12g fiber | 40g net carbohydrate

Nutrition Facts Totals for Day 6: *2,127 calories | 149g fat | 85g protein | 65g carbohydrate | 19g fiber | 46g net carbohydrate*

DAY 7

Breakfast · 12 ounces coffee, black

Lunch · 1 serving Crispy Spiced Chicken Tenders (page 148)

· ½ cup steamed broccoli with 2 tablespoons butter

· Side salad with lettuce, olives, celery, and olive oil

· 8 ounces water

883 calories | 81g fat | 28g protein | 15g carbohydrate | 11g fiber | 4g net carbohydrate

Dinner · 1 serving Peanut Chicken Kabobs (page 155)

· 1 serving Sweet Potato Curry (page 168) served with 1 serving Paneer (page 136)

· 1 serving Indian Spiced "Corn" Bread (page 132)

1,245 calories | 75g fat | 89g protein | 60g carbohydrate | 16g fiber | 44g net carbohydrate

Nutrition Facts Totals for Day 7: *2,128 calories | 156g fat | 117g protein | 75g carbohydrate | 27g fiber | 48g net carbohydrate*

Key Takeaways

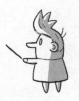

1. Eat whole foods. Base your meals around quality protein and fats with a moderate amount of carbohydrates for variety and pleasure.

2. Avoid processed foods, gluten-containing grains, inflammatory oils, and factory-farmed meat whenever possible.

3. Incorporate some aspect of intermittent fasting into your routine. The specifics are less important than the intent.

Chapter Six

Diet Is Not Enough:

Lifestyle Considerations

You've probably heard the phrase "you can't out-exercise a bad diet." Well, the reverse is true as well. You can't out-diet a bad lifestyle. And by lifestyle, I don't just mean physical activity. While that is absolutely an important part of it, it is also not enough. I know it is a bummer that I'm telling you there is a lot more to wellness than diet and exercise. Sorry, but that's the truth as I understand it; we are complicated biological creatures with the additional complication of having complex emotional needs.

I consider there to be five factors of health: diet, physical activity, stress management, sleep, and a sense of purpose/belonging. We'll discuss each one (other than diet) in this chapter. Think of the five factors as a stool: four legs and a seat. You need all of them together to have a good, sturdy stool.

You need to mind all these factors even if your only goal is weight loss (which it should not be), because several wellness practitioners have reported seeing many of their clients unable to lose the weight they want until getting their other lifestyle factors sorted out. And this makes perfect sense. Any one of these factors being out of balance can change the way your body partitions fuel and the overall metabolic environment of your body.

While I want to give you some broad strokes of what I understand to be best practices in these areas, keep in mind that I'm a dietitian and these other factors are outside my scope of practice. If you want to learn more about any of the four pillars other than diet, check Resources on page 194 for some good books and professionals in those fields.

Physical Activity

Before we talk about the benefits of appropriate physical activity, let's get a misconception out of the way. The idea that we exercise to burn calories to stay lean is, frankly, ludicrous. Exercise is not a weight-loss tool. This statement is very well supported by scientific evidence and has been for years. While exercise without diet intervention can produce modest weight loss, it is not as much as you would mathematically predict. Not only is it very difficult to actually burn a significant amount of calories with a realistic exercise routine, but our bodies don't appear to burn calories during exercise in the way that we expect. So, like with calorie counts of food, you're somewhat working blind if you are trying to offset some food with some exercise. Additionally, whether it is psychological or physiological, people appear to participate in something called compensatory behaviors when they are exercising for weight loss. These compensatory behaviors can manifest as a spontaneous increase in energy intake (you eat more without noticing) or as a spontaneous reduction of energy (you move less for the rest of the day). Either way, it's a wash.

The reason we still collectively regard exercise as a weight-loss tool is because the processed food industry and almost every mainstream health organization still maintains that weight management is about "eating less and moving more." Without getting too deep into any conspiracy theories, I will note that this ideology is beneficial to the processed food industry. If the reason so many Americans are overweight or obese is because we eat too much and move too little, there is no responsibility to be had by the industry.

I've told you what exercise is not. Now let me tell you what it is: a magic, anti-aging, injury- and disease-preventing, mood-boosting wellness tool. Though I understand that all our lives are hectic and it can be difficult to find the time and motivation for exercise, it should be a non-negotiable part of your routine.

The USDA's guidelines for physical activity for Americans are that we participate in two and a half hours of moderate activity or an hour and fifteen minutes of vigorous aerobic activity per week, and at least two sessions of resistance training that engages all muscle groups per week. Amazingly, I mostly agree with the USDA on this one. However, I think the priorities should be reversed. My understanding of the evidence is that, in terms of bang-for-buck, resistance training should be the priority. Both styles of exercise are useful for wellness and health but resistance training has the added benefit of increasing muscle mass to a greater extent in less time.

Increasing muscle mass means increasing glucose disposal and therefore carbohydrate tolerance. By that, I mean the greater amount of muscle mass you have, the more carbohydrate your body can effectively use before overwhelming the system and becoming a problem. Muscle mass is also a priority for healthy aging. The age-related loss of lean muscle mass is associated with increased falls, negative clinical outcomes, and serious debility. And don't worry, strength training does not necessarily need to mean deadlifts and squats and getting swole. It simply means incorporating strength training into your routine.

I only feel comfortable giving you broad-stroke recommendations for what type of program you should follow in regard to strength training and recommend that in the beginning you work with a qualified personal trainer to make sure your form is correct and the program you are following is appropriate for your goals. You do not necessarily need to use free weights or flip tires to get a workout that is hard enough to be beneficial. You can use machines, resistance bands, or even your own body weight to great success. The important part is that you are engaging all your body's muscle groups and that you are stressing them sufficiently to induce growth and strengthening.

You should also incorporate aerobic exercise into your daily routine. There are many ways to incorporate this type of activity. You can bike or run or swim or hike or climb, etc. An important thing to note is that research indicates that you do not have to spend hours jogging or cycling to glean significant benefit. It looks like you can trade time for intensity. Researchers randomized 55 non-athlete college students into three groups and tracked their response to three different training routines. One group participated in low-intensity, steady-state exercise for 20 minutes, one group did 13 moderate-intensity intervals of 30 seconds work and 60 seconds active rest for a total of 20 minutes, and a final group performed 8 sets of high-intensity intervals for a total of 4 minutes. At the end of the study, all three groups showed similar increases in aerobic and anaerobic work capacity. So, all three groups got stronger and gained endurance. This study had another interesting and salient finding: All three of the groups reported enjoying their workout less and less over the course of the study.

This brings me to my next point: Don't do exercise you don't like. There are so many ways to get physical activity and a big part of their point is to make you feel better on a daily basis. If you hate the form of exercise you are doing, it defeats the purpose a bit. Of course, there will be days you don't want to do *anything*, but if you always dread the workout, you should try out a different kind of physical activity. The important thing is that you're doing something and that you're doing it on a regular basis.

"The best diet is the one you can follow" is a saying that I wholeheartedly endorse. The same is true of exercise. Even if all the science in the world were telling you that Russian kettlebell training, for example, is the best possible type of exercise, it would be meaningless to your life if you hate Russian kettlebell training and skip out on it more often than not.

Stress Management

Stress in the modern world is pretty detached from the stress our bodies likely evolved to face. Our physiological stress response of increased heart rate, increased levels of cortisol and norepinephrine (adrenaline), and an increased blood glucose level are much more appropriate for running away from a predator than for worrying about how to pay our bills every day.

That stress response was appropriate when stress was an intermittent and acute experience. Now most of us enjoy lives relatively free of physically stressful situations, but we've traded that physical security for an increase in psychological stress. We worry about darn near everything. Some of the things we worry about are reasonable, like paying our bills and what we're going to do when the zombie apocalypse comes, but many of the things we worry about are not, from a survival perspective, worth the physiological cost.

The types of stress we encounter on a continuous basis have been associated with dysfunctional eating and obesity, heart disease, systemic inflammation and increased frequency of illness, and even lower capacity for empathy. And aside from the bad things that chronic stress can do to your health, it is just no fun. I have heard it described as mental background noise or the mean little voice that lives in your head. No matter which metaphor you use to describe the constant, low-level stress we all live with, you need to take steps to better handle it.

I don't think that stress reduction is all that realistic in our society. Everyone has bills, social pressures, and emotional baggage of their own. Nothing can be done about most of the sources of stress in our lives. For most people, it makes more sense to attempt to improve our reaction to stress rather than to try to reduce our amount of stress. Instead of stress reduction, let's call it stress mitigation, stress management, or (my favorite) distress tolerance. The idea is to make our emotional capabilities and ourselves more robust and resilient.

The best way that I've found to increase distress tolerance is meditation.

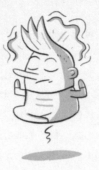

Meditation has been shown to be beneficial for the reduction of stress-related anxiety in healthy individuals but may also offer some relief to those with more debilitating levels of stress. There have been a number of studies showing a reduction in self-reported stress, anxiety, and feelings of panic when people with post-traumatic stress syndrome receive mindfulness training and maintain a mindfulness practice. There is evidence that a mindfulness practice can slow age-related cognitive decline and improve the memory and cognition of people with dementia. It even looks like a regular meditative practice can help you get control of some disordered eating behaviors like binge and emotional eating.

Meditation is simply the practice of controlling your attention. It is like exercising the cognitive muscles that allow you to focus. Just as you need to put the time and effort into building your physical muscles, you need to put the time into building your cognitive muscles. I think of it as a way to reduce the background noise of my consciousness. It does not reduce the emotions and distracting thoughts you experience, it just allows you to choose how you react to them a little better.

Think of it like this: It is the difference between being inside the drum of a washing machine on the high cycle and standing over the drum observing it. Inside the drum, you are being tossed around, sloshed up, soaked, and mixed up with everything else. Imagine trying to focus on anything in that situation. In the other scenario, you can look down on the chaos of all those clothes in the washing machine drum and choose where to focus your attention. You can track a red sock as it sloshes around, you can watch the perimeter of the drum rotate, or you can watch the whole load, not focusing on any one aspect. Though it is only a difference of a few inches of perspective, sometimes that can make all the difference.

I'm not going to give you any direct instructions for a routine to follow because there are many different methods of meditation and they all work. There are a variety of programs and applications to help you make meditation a part of your life. Check the Resources section for a list of apps and books if you are looking for a place to start.

Sleep

I hinted at the importance of sleep earlier, but I'll reiterate: Sleep is really, really important. In fact, if I had to pick one of the five pillars that you *need* for health and wellness, it would be sleep. You can have all the other pillars sorted, but if the amount or quality of the sleep you're getting is inadequate, you will still feel awful and be at a higher risk of illness. Sleep is essential for tissue and muscle recovery, mental clarity, mood, immune function, and ability to make it through a day.

Inadequate sleep is associated with fat gain and muscle loss regardless of caloric intake, and it promotes increased intake of lower-quality food. That means if you're sleep deprived, your body will tell you eat more in total, specifically more crappy food, and it will store more of the calories that you eat as fat instead of muscle. That's a pretty bad deal.

Though it is nearly impossible to study in a definitive way, there is good theoretical basis for the idea that inadequate sleep actually makes you age worse. That is, inadequate sleep over a long period will increase the number and types of genes being expressed that are associated with aging, increased tissue breakdown and degradation, increased inflammation, and decreased cognitive ability.

Additionally, you will feel pain more acutely when you're sleep deprived. You don't want to be an overweight, overeating, under-muscled, prematurely aged, unthinking, inflamed, and pained person, do you?

There are two considerations when discussing sleep: quantity and quality. Sleep quantity is the total amount of time spent sleeping. The amount you need for optimal function will vary, but on average it is between 7 and 8 hours. Sleep quality is a more subjective measure. The quality of your sleep has to do with how restorative it feels, how long it takes you to fall asleep, how many times you wake throughout the night, how long it takes to fall back asleep if you wake, and how long you spend in the different stages of sleep.

You need to be mindful of both factors for optimal sleep. Let's talk about a concept called sleep hygiene that can help you get better sleep. Sleep hygiene is the idea that there are some best practices involving sleep timing, light exposure, temperature, nutrient timing, and noise control.

Sleep Timing

Sleep timing has to do with the idea of circadian rhythms. We all have a sleep-wake cycle that follows a roughly 24-hour routine. Despite the popular idea that there are "morning people" and "night owls," studies show that everyone is likely a "when the sun is up" type of person, if they are removed from artificial sources of light and sound. This means that as far as we know, the optimal sleep-wake cycle should track pretty closely with natural light.

As far as specific timing, you start by trying to build a routine that lets you be asleep (not in bed–actually asleep) for 7.5 hours. If you need to adjust this timing up or down, work in 90-minute blocks. The reason for this recommendation has to do with sleep cycles. When asleep, we cycle through four sleep stages: 1, 2, 3, and rapid eye movement (REM). Think of these cycles as points along a V. Stage 1 is at the top of one side of the V and REM is on top at the other side. The valley of the V would be stages 2 and 3. We cycle from stage 1 to REM about every 90 minutes and then start over. Stages 1 and REM are relatively light stages of sleep, and 2 and 3 are deeper. If you are awakened during one of the lighter stages, you will feel more rested and alert, but if you are awakened during stage 2 or 3, it is more likely that you will feel groggy and terrible. To increase the chance that you will be working with these cycles and not against them, try to time your waking in one of the lighter stages. If you know when you need to be awake, simply count backward from that time in 90 minute increments. Optimally, you want to get five or six of these increments–7.5 or 9 hours. Account for the amount of time it will take you to fall asleep in this estimation. Supposedly, it takes 14 minutes on average for people to fall asleep, but this is a very rough average and it can take more time for you. This is an area where self-knowledge is helpful.

Light Exposure

Blue light wavelength exposure tells your neurobiological systems that it is time to be awake. Unfortunately, all the traditional artificial light sources we are exposed to in our modern world include this blue wavelength. Try to avoid blue light exposure starting 2 to 3 hours before you want to be asleep. There are now a variety of apps available to block the blue wavelength of light on your devices. The latest versions of Android and iOS even have native settings to do this. You can find low-light or amber-light nightlights to use for reading and you can even get blue light-blocking glasses to wear in the evenings.

For many people, limiting blue light exposure will be enough, but for some, any light exposure is distracting on a psychological level. It can interfere with falling asleep initially but also make it harder to fall asleep if they wake in the night. Some people find benefit in making their rooms cave-like in terms of light by shutting out lights from electronics like humidifiers and digital clocks and letting no light in from the windows. Blackout curtains can be an extreme but useful tool.

Temperature

Part of your body's regulation of your wake-sleep cycle has to do with core body temperature, which should naturally lower while you are sleeping and gradually rise as you get closer to waking. The commonly repeated recommendation is to keep your room temperature somewhere between 60°F and 65°F to help your body with this process. However, try as I might, I could not find this recommendation backed by any white-coat science. What we can prove is that temperature fluctuation matters a great deal to sleep quality and that lower temperatures tend to be correlated with more time spent in the deep sleep cycles. I would start with a cooler temperature in the 60°F to 65°F range and tweak up or down based on your subjective experience of sleep.

Nutrient Timing

By nutrient timing, I mean two things: avoid caffeine exposure in a way that makes sense for you and avoid late evening meals.

As we already discussed, caffeine is metabolized in wildly different ways based on several factors. I think it is worth trying to stop drinking caffeine after noon for about a week and see if you notice any difference in how wakeful and rested you feel in the mornings. If you're getting enough (quantity) of sleep but still feel hit by a truck in the mornings, it is likely your sleep quality is cruddy, and it is likely caffeine is a factor.

Additionally, you should avoid late evening meals (or, put differently, meals within 2 to 3 hours of when you would like to be asleep) to help promote the naturalization of your circadian rhythm. Of course, if you're following my recommendations from the previous chapter and incorporating some longer fasting times into your daily routine, this should be easy-peasy.

Noise Control

This one is obvious: You need it to be quiet in your sleep space. White noise like a fan or ocean sounds is probably okay.

***

If you sort all these factors out and are still having issues falling or staying asleep, it may be useful to incorporate some supplemental tools. Chamomile tea has some evidence of efficacy, as do melatonin and the neurotransmitter precursor 5-HTP. Experiment and figure out what works for you.

A note about some of the other methods people use to get to sleep, like alcohol and pharmaceuticals: Don't. Alcohol may help you feel drowsy and fall asleep but it actually worsens the quality of your sleep. You're robbing Peter to pay Paul. Popular sleep aids like Ambien have a different problem. They have been shown to effectively knock you out quickly. But that appears to be literally what is happening: You are being knocked *unconscious* but you are not *asleep*. They are not the same thing. The biggest difference is memory consolidation and effective shutdown of certain brain functions. That's why some of the side effects of these types of drugs are things like sleep-eating and sleep-sex. Oh, and they might increase your risk of dying.

Sense of Purpose/Belonging

This one may seem obvious, but it is an issue for most of us on some level. Believing that your actions matter and that the sum total of your life has some meaning on some level is certainly better than the alternative. Though it is very hard to study conclusively, researchers believe that having a sense of purpose and belonging to a group may be a determining factor in overall health and have an effect on longevity.

Researchers have found that the greater a person believes their purpose in life to be, the lower their risk of cardiovascular event. That makes perfect sense to me because if you believe that you have a purpose and are working toward or even fulfilling that purpose, it is likely that you are experiencing less chronic systemic stress and therefore overall inflammation. Somewhat surprisingly, a sense of purpose is also associated with greater measures of physical capability during aging. People who reported higher levels of purpose and belonging in life were found to have greater grip strength and gait speed. Both of those measures are understood to be predictors of overall health in older individuals. Additionally, when blue zones, areas identified to have more people living to 100 or greater than in the general population, are studied, a sense of purpose and community belonging are consistently found to be part of what makes them special.

I understand that "find a purpose and sense of belonging" as a recommendation is about as useful as "learn to fly!" But, the evidence says what it says, and here we are. You have a better shot of being happy and healthy if you feel like you are a part of something larger than yourself. The good news is that there are many ways to do this.

Participation in organized religion is associated with a sense of purpose in life but becoming religiously oriented is not exactly something you can choose to do. So, if you feel inclined to any type of religious participation, have at it. If you are not religiously inclined, helping other people is a proven way to develop a sense of purpose that rivals that of religious belief.

Not all helping is equal, though. To get the sense-of-purpose benefit of helping others, you need to be participating voluntarily (so no court-ordered helping!) and the people you are helping should be relatively unknown to you. Helping friends and family is not associated with the same levels of purpose as helping strangers. Also, getting paid for helping strangers does not appear to count. So, help people you don't know and do it because you want to help people.

You Are Worth the Effort

Really. You are.

Getting your diet and all these lifestyle factors in line is no easy feat. It requires a lot of work and consistent effort. However, getting these things sorted will make you feel better in every moment of every day. I'm not exaggerating the power of dedicating the time and energy to legitimately take care of yourself. You will feel a difference in each moment of your day. The good things in your day will be richer and deeper and the bad things will be easier to accept. You may even come to see things you currently regard as bad things differently. It is difficult to overstate how profoundly your perspective can change just from accepting that you are worth some time and effort.

In addition, you'll feel stronger, more refreshed, more centered, and like you are a part of something larger than yourself. But it really starts with just accepting that you deserve to feel those things. Many of us accept our own status quo because, on some level, we feel like that is the most we deserve to expect. That is nonsense. None of us deserve to feel less than our best.

Main Takeaways

1. True health is about much more than diet. Diet is not enough.

2. You also have to mind your physical activity, stress tolerance, sleep, and sense of purpose.

3. You are worth the effort.

Chapter Seven

Recipes

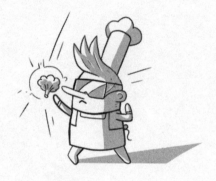

Bread

Everything Bagel (Flavored) Biscuits

To get the tough-on-the-outside, chewy-on-the-inside texture we associate with traditional bagels, you boil the dough for a few minutes prior to baking. This allows for the crust to be a little bit cooked before it goes in the oven, which somewhat protects the inside from the heat. I tried a whole bunch of different methods and I've determined that it is not possible (at least in a home kitchen with normal ingredients) to produce the same bagel texture with keto-friendly ingredients. You should have seen the mess I made trying to boil a few varieties of keto dough.

Even though the texture is not quite perfect, the flavor of these biscuits is amazing. Once you slather them with a generous helping of cream cheese, you really won't miss that extra bit of chewiness. These make for a fantastic breakfast or lunch on the go.

Prep Time: 5 minutes | *Cook Time:* 15 to 20 minutes | *Yield:* 6 servings

4 tablespoons butter, melted and divided

1 tablespoon coconut butter, melted

3 eggs

1 teaspoon poppy seeds

2 teaspoons dried oregano

½ cup plus 1 tablespoon almond flour

1 tablespoon coconut flour

2 teaspoons baking powder

1 teaspoon onion powder

1 teaspoon garlic powder

1 teaspoon salt

2 teaspoons sesame seeds

2 teaspoons dehydrated onion flakes

1. Preheat the oven to 350°F.

2. In a large mixing bowl, combine 3 tablespoons of melted butter and coconut butter. Mix well.

3. Add eggs, poppy seeds, and oregano to mixture. Mix well.

4. Sift in the almond flour, coconut flour, baking powder, onion powder, garlic powder, and salt. Mix well.

5. Grease a bagel pan or a muffin tin with the remaining 1 tablespoon of melted butter. With a muffin tin, you won't get that distinctive bagel shape, but they will still be delicious. Divide the batter evenly among your bagel or muffin wells. Sprinkle the sesame seeds and onion flakes on top of each.

6. Bake for 15 to 20 minutes until the edges of the biscuits are brown. Let cool before attempting to cut and spread anything on them.

Nutrition per Serving
180 calories | 17g fat | 6g protein | 4g carbohydrate | 2g fiber | 2g net carbohydrate

Wonder (fully Like White) Bread

I really love using a lot spices in my keto bread recipes because, well, flavors are awesome. But, sometimes you just want that almost-nothing taste of Wonder Bread that many of us grew up with. This bread is great for toasting and slathering in butter, or for making a good old-fashioned PB&J (with no-sugar-added peanut butter and mashed berries instead of jelly, of course). It is also a great base for making garlic bread. Just toast and add some garlic and herbed butter.

I recommend adding yeast to this recipe to give it a more bread-like flavor, but it is not essential. Similarly, the cream of tartar and xanthan gum improve the texture of the recipe, but both ingredients are optional.

Prep Time: 15 minutes | Cook Time: 35 to 40 minutes | Yield: 8 to 10 servings

1 ½ cups superfine almond flour

1 teaspoon salt

2 teaspoons baking powder

¼ teaspoon xanthan gum, optional

1 tablespoon dry active yeast, optional

6 eggs, whites and yolks separated

4 tablespoons butter, melted

⅛ teaspoon cream of tartar, optional

1. Preheat the oven to 325°F and line a bread pan with parchment paper, allowing some to stick out of the top. This will make removal of the loaf much easier.

2. If you are not using superfine almond flour, add your almond flour to the work bowl of a food processor and pulse until it is as fine as you can make it.

3. Add the almond flour, salt, baking powder, xanthan gum, yeast, if using, egg yolks, and butter to the work bowl of a food processor and pulse until very well combined. You will have to scrape the sides down a few times.

4. In a separate bowl, add the cream of tartar, if using, to the egg whites and beat them until very stiff peaks are formed.

5. Mix about half of the stiff egg whites into the almond flour mixture and pulse until just combined. Don't overmix.

6. Using a rubber spatula, carefully fold the almond flour mixture into the remaining egg whites just until you don't see any more streaks of white. Your bread gets its height and structure from the stiff egg whites and the more you work this mixture, the less structure it will have.

7. Transfer the batter into your lined bread pan and bake in the oven for 35 to 40 minutes. Allow to cool completely before slicing.

Nutrition per Serving

200 calories | 18g fat | 8g protein | 4g carbohydrate | 2g fiber | 2g net carbohydrate

Cheddar Jalapeno "Corn" Bread

Cornbread is so iconic that if you are used to having it with something (ahem, chili), then you *really* miss it when it's not there. I experimented with several variations before landing on this combination of ingredients and method in order to replicate the coarse and somewhat heavy texture of Southern cornbread.

Prep Time: 5 minutes | Cook Time: 12 to 15 minutes | Yield: 6 servings

1 cup almond flour

½ teaspoon salt

½ teaspoon baking powder

2 eggs

1 cup shredded cheddar cheese

2 tablespoons sour cream

¼ cup diced jalapenos (fresh or pickled)

butter, for greasing skillet

1. Preheat the oven to 350°F and thoroughly grease a 10-inch cast-iron skillet with butter.

2. In a large bowl, mix the almond flour, salt, and baking powder.

3. In a separate bowl, mix the eggs, cheese, sour cream, and jalapenos.

4. Fold the almond flour mixture into the cheese mixture.

5. Pour the batter into your skillet and smooth it out. Bake for 12 to 15 minutes, until firm and just starting to brown. Let cool then slice into 6 equal portions.

Nutrition per Serving
240 calories | 20g fat | 11g protein | 5g carbohydrate | 2g fiber | 3g net carbohydrate

Sweet Potato Buttermilk Drop Biscuits

These biscuits are dense and so densely flavorful. They are like moist fall-flavored bombs. You may obtain your sweet potato puree from any source you please. I like to get a big sweet potato, roast it in the oven at 375°F for about an hour, then scoop out the insides. You can also find sweet potato canned.

Prep Time: 5 minutes | *Cook Time:* 15 to 20 minutes | *Yield:* 6 servings

1 cup almond flour

1 cup sweet potato puree

1 teaspoon baking soda

1 teaspoon baking powder

½ teaspoon cinnamon

½ teaspoon nutmeg

½ teaspoon salt

¼ cup buttermilk

4 tablespoons butter, diced into ¼-inch cubes and chilled

1. Preheat the oven to 425°F.

2. In the work bowl of a food processor or stand mixer, combine the almond flour, sweet potato puree, baking soda, baking powder, cinnamon, nutmeg, and salt. Mix until smooth.

3. Add the buttermilk and mix again.

4. Take the butter out of the fridge and use immediately. Add the chilled butter cubes a little at a time, folding the dough. You're trying to get them pretty evenly distributed without allowing them to melt or get broken up too much.

5. Using a big spoon, plop 6 equal-sized blobs onto a greased baking pan. Allow a few inches between each. They won't spread all that much, but there will be some creep.

6. Bake for 15 to 20 minutes until the biscuits start to brown.

Nutrition per Serving

220 calories | 17g fat | 6g protein | 9g carbohydrate | 3g fiber | 6g net carbohydrate

Perfect Keto Muffins

I don't usually title things "perfect" because it feels like hype and nonsense. However, these really are the perfect keto muffins. I tested, and if I don't tell a person, they cannot tell they are keto. That's usually my measure for true success for a low-carb baked good. Otherwise—and this applies to some of my creations—they are not great, but just good enough.

These muffins are great.

They actually started life as a waffle batter I was trying to perfect. After about a week of varying-quality waffles for dinner every night, I had a recipe I was happy with. Then I calculated the nutrition info—nearly 1,000 calories per waffle! So I decided to break the batter into smaller servings to make it a little less ridiculous. After a little more tweaking, the perfect keto muffins were born.

I also consider them to be a base. While they are great on their own, they will also be great if you add blueberries or cheddar cheese or even blueberries and cheddar cheese. These are highly customizable.

Prep Time: 5 minutes | Cook Time: 20 minutes | Yield: 6 servings

2 eggs

1 ounce softened cream cheese

¼ cup almond flour

2 tablespoons coconut flour

2 tablespoons flaxseed meal

2 tablespoons smooth peanut butter

2 tablespoons coconut oil

2 tablespoons unsweetened soy or almond milk

1 teaspoon vanilla extract

½ teaspoon baking powder

½ teaspoon salt

1½ tablespoons steel cut oats, divided

1. Preheat the oven to 350°F and line a muffin tin with 6 muffin cups.

2. Crack the eggs into a large bowl and whisk vigorously until they lighten in color and are frothy.

3. Add all ingredients except for ½ tablespoon oats to the bowl. Mix until smooth.

4. Equally divide the batter into the muffin cups and sprinkle a few oats on top of each muffin.

5. Bake for 20 minutes. Let the muffins cool before consuming. Store on the counter in an airtight container for up to 4 days.

Nutrition per Serving
175 calories | 6g protein | 14g fat | 6g carbohydrate | 2g fiber | 4g net carbohydrate

Tortilla Chips

Every once in a while you just *need* chips. Whether it is because you want a big ole mess of nachos or you need something for scooping melted queso into your mouth other than a spoon, these will do the trick. They are salty and crunchy like good chips should be. Don't try to use them in tortilla soup–it won't work. Do use them to eat hummus or Buffalo Chicken Dip (page 177).

Prep Time: 5 minutes | Cook Time: 10 minutes |
Yield: 8 servings

1 ½ cups almond flour

1 teaspoon cumin

1 teaspoon chili powder

½ teaspoon coriander

¼ teaspoon cayenne pepper

1 teaspoon granulated salt

2 teaspoons fresh ground pepper

1 egg, beaten

½ cup mozzarella cheese

3 tablespoons ghee or lard, for frying

1. In a large bowl, combine the almond flour, cumin, chili powder, coriander, cayenne pepper, and granulated salt.

2. Add the egg and mix well.

3. In a separate bowl, melt the mozzarella cheese by microwaving it in 30-second increments or over a double boiler.

4. Combine the almond flour mixture and melted mozzarella cheese. Using a wooden spoon or your hands (careful, it may be hot), mix very well until a homogeneous dough is formed.

5. Put the dough between 2 pieces of parchment and roll it flat, until you have a very thin sheet of dough. It should be as thin as possible, without it separating when lifted. Slice the dough into roughly 1 ½-inch-wide triangles.

6. Heat the ghee or lard over medium-high heat in a heavy-bottomed pan like a cast-iron skillet.

7. Fry your dough triangles for about a minute on each side or until crispy and ever so slightly browned. Transfer the chips onto some paper towels and pat off the excess oil.

Nutrition per Serving

155 calories | 13g fat | 7g protein | 5g carbohydrate | 2g fiber | 3g net carbohydrate

Pizza Crust

Prep Time: 20 minutes | *Cook Time:* 25 minutes | *Yield:* 6 to 8 slices

2 ½ cups shredded mozzarella

2 ounces cream cheese

1 ½ cups almond flour

½ teaspoon baking powder

¼ teaspoon xanthan gum

½ tablespoon dried oregano

½ teaspoon salt

½ teaspoon garlic powder

½ teaspoon crushed red pepper

½ cup warm water

1 (0.25-ounce) packet instant yeast

1 egg

1. Preheat the oven to 350°F.

2. Combine the mozzarella and cream cheese in large microwave-safe bowl. Microwave in 30-second increments, stirring between each, until smooth and combined.

3. Combine the almond flour, baking powder, xanthan gum, oregano, salt, garlic powder, and crushed red pepper. For best results, sift the almond flour, baking powder, and xanthan gum into the bowl. You will get a texture closer to glutinous bread this way.

4. Combine the water and yeast in a small bowl and stir.

5. Add the yeast, water, and egg to the almond flour mixture. Stir until well mixed, roll into a ball, and let rest for 10 minutes.

6. Transfer the dough to a parchment paper-lined baking sheet and roll into a circle or rectangle.

7. Bake for 15 minutes. Remove the crust from the oven, add desired sauce and toppings, and return to the oven for additional 10 minutes.

8. Remove the pizza from the oven. Let cool, and slice into desired number of slices.

Nutrition per Serving

96 calories | 8g fat | 4g protein | 2g carbohydrate | 1g fiber | 1g net carbohydrate

Indian Spiced "Corn" Bread

Traditionally, this dish is made with chickpea flour and it is steamed instead of baked. The result is a very moist and dense bread that is somehow also fluffy. This version is closer to American-style cornbread, but the spice mixture brings the same flavor profile as the traditional version. Same amazing, nuanced taste, much fewer carbs!

Prep Time: 5 minutes | Cook Time: 12 to 15 minutes | Yield: 6 servings

1 cup almond flour

½ teaspoon salt

½ teaspoon ground cumin

½ teaspoon ground coriander seed

½ teaspoon chili powder

½ teaspoon baking powder

2 eggs

1 cup shredded mozzarella cheese

2 tablespoons sour cream

2 teaspoons mustard seeds

½ cup fresh cilantro, chopped

2 Thai green chiles, sliced lengthwise and deseeded

1. Preheat the oven to 350°F and thoroughly grease a 10-inch cast-iron skillet with butter.

2. In a large bowl, mix the almond flour, salt, cumin, coriander seed, chili powder, and baking powder.

3. In a separate bowl, mix the eggs, cheese, and sour cream. Fold the almond flour mixture into the cheese mixture.

4. Pour the batter into your skillet and smooth it out. Bake for 12 to 15 minutes until the bread is firm and just starting to brown.

5. Remove the bread from the oven and distribute mustard seeds, cilantro, and green chiles across the top.

6. Let cool, then slice into 6 equal portions.

Nutrition per Serving

240 calories | 20g fat | 11g protein | 4g carbohydrate | 2g fiber | 2g net carbohydrate

Fat Head Bread

If you have spent any time at all looking at low-carb bread-like recipes online, you have seen some version of Fat Head Bread. To my knowledge, no one knows who developed this recipe, but it has become a favorite of the keto community. With good reason. It yields a dense and versatile bread that can be used for muffins, sandwiches, pizza crust, and more. This is intended as a base recipe to be customized as you see fit.

Prep Time: 5 minutes | Cook Time: 20 to 25 minutes | Yield: 8 slices

2 ½ cups shredded mozzarella

2 ounces cream cheese

1 ½ cups almond flour

½ teaspoon baking powder

½ teaspoon salt

2 eggs

1. Preheat the oven to 350°F.

2. Combine the mozzarella and cream cheese in large microwave-safe bowl. Microwave in 30-second increments, stirring between each, until smooth and combined.

3. Combine the almond flour, baking powder, and salt. For best results, sift the almond flour and baking powder into the bowl.

4. Add the eggs to the almond flour mixture, and stir until well mixed.

5. Transfer the dough to a loaf pan. Bake for 20 to 25 minutes until the top starts to brown.

6. Remove the bread from the oven. Let cool, slice into desired number of slices.

Nutrition per Serving
81 calories | 8g fat | 4g protein | 2g carbohydrate | 1g fiber | 1g net carbohydrate

Cheese

Crème Fraîche

You can think of crème fraîche as a slightly tangy soft cheese with a rich mouthfeel, or you can think of it as I do: Heavy Whipping Cream Yogurt. This is really the perfect thing for a keto diet because it is high fat, almost no carb, and just heavenly. It's also crazy simple to make.

Prep Time: 1 minute, plus rest time |
Yield: 8 servings

8 ounces heavy whipping cream

1 tablespoon cultured buttermilk

1. Combine heavy whipping cream and buttermilk in a glass container. Give it a stir. I usually use a pint mason jar.

2. Cover the glass container with a clean towel.

3. Leave the mixture at room temperature for 8 to 24 hours, depending on how thick and how tangy you want it to be. The longer it sits, the tangier it will be.

4. Seal the container and store in the refrigerator for up to 10 days.

Nutrition per Serving
107 calories | 1g protein | 11g fat | 1g carbohydrate | 0g fiber | 1g net carbohydrate

Paneer

You'll notice that this recipe is pretty close to the Cottage Cheese recipe on page 140. That's because paneer is basically pressed cottage cheese. Paneer is a traditional Indian cheese with a really delightful texture. You can use it anytime you would like a soft-but-solid mild cheese. It's good in curries and works well in salads, too.

Prep Time: 1 minute | Cook Time: 45 to 50 minutes | Yield: 4 (½-cup) servings

1 gallon whole milk

½ cup heavy whipping cream

¾ cup lemon juice

½ teaspoon salt

1. Pour the milk and heavy whipping cream into a large pot and heat over medium-low heat until it reaches roughly 120°F, or until it starts to steam.

2. Remove the milk from the heat and pour in the lemon juice. Stir gently for 1 to 2 minutes. The curds should begin to separate from the whey.

3. Cover and leave at room temperature for about 30 minutes.

4. Line a colander with cheesecloth. It is best to use a colander with a mostly flat bottom since you'll be pressing the cheese. I like to stack about 4 sheets of cheesecloth.

5. Pour the curds and whey mixture into the cheesecloth-lined colander. Rinse under cold water for 2 to 3 minutes to get all of the lemon taste out.

6. Add salt, and mix.

7. Fold up the edges of your cheesecloth to make a neat little cheese square.

8. Put something heavy, like a cast-iron skillet, on top of the cheese square while it is still in the colander and let it press for about an hour.

9. Remove your heavy thing, peel the cheesecloth off, transfer your paneer into a storage container, and store in the refrigerator for 2 to 3 days.

Nutrition per Serving

120 calories | 5g fat | 14g protein | 4g carbohydrate | 0g fiber | 4g net carbohydrate

Baked Brie Cheese

Brie is pretty fantastic on its own, but baking it inside of a Fat Head Bread shell makes for a creamy, melty, nuanced treat. It is very easy to make and can serve as a great party food or dinner.

Prep Time: 30 minutes | Cook Time: 30 minutes | Yield: 12 servings

1 recipe Fat Head Bread (page 134)

1 (8-ounce) round Brie cheese

¼ cup slivered almonds

1. Preheat the oven to 325°F.

2. Prepare Fat Head Bread as described, but roll into a 6- to 8-inch circle instead of baking in a loaf pan.

3. Place the Brie in the center of your dough circle and fold the edges over the top of the cheese, fully encasing the cheese.

4. Bake for 25 minutes. Remove the Brie from the oven, sprinkle slivered almonds on top, and return to the oven for another 5 minutes.

5. Remove the Brie from the oven. Let cool for 3 to 5 minutes before cutting into 12 equal portions.

Nutrition per Serving
158 calories | 14g fat | 8g protein | 3g carbohydrate | 2g fiber | 1g net carbohydrate

Mediterranean Marinated Goat Cheese

My first book was *The Ketogenic Mediterranean Diet* and while writing it I developed quite a soft spot for the fantastic blend of spices associated with Mediterranean foods. Marinated goat cheese is wonderfully rich and creamy. When combined with high-quality olive oil and fresh spices, it becomes a flavor explosion the likes of which you cannot match. This recipe is a great addition to salads or served on top of a nice steak. You can also reuse the marinade, adding spices as needed.

Prep Time: 5 minutes, plus rest time |
Yield: 6 servings

6 ounces goat cheese, sliced into 1-ounce rounds

1 cup extra virgin olive oil

½ tablespoon black peppercorns

1 tablespoon finely chopped fresh basil

1 teaspoon dried oregano

1 teaspoon dried thyme

1 teaspoon dried parsley

1. Mix the oil and spices until the spices are evenly distributed in the oil.

2. Combine all ingredients in a shallow glass container with a lid. It should be shallow enough to ensure the goat cheese medallions are covered by the oil and spice mixture.

3. Place in the refrigerator and let marinate for a minimum of an hour before serving.

Nutrition per Serving
155 calories | 15g fat | 5g protein | 0g carbohydrate | 0g fiber | 0g net carbohydrate

Cottage Cheese

Prep Time: 1 minute | Cook Time: 45 to 50 minutes |
Yield: 4 (½-cup) servings

1 gallon whole milk

¾ cup white vinegar

½ cup heavy
whipping cream

salt, to taste

1. Pour the milk into a large pot and heat over medium-low heat until it reaches roughly 120°F, or until it starts to steam.

2. Remove the milk from the heat and pour in the vinegar. Stir gently for 1 to 2 minutes. The curds should begin to separate from the whey.

3. Cover and leave at room temperature for about 30 minutes.

4. Line a colander with cheesecloth. It is best to use a colander with a mostly flat bottom since you'll be pressing the cheese. I like to stack about 4 sheets of cheesecloth.

5. Pour the curds and whey mixture into the cheesecloth-lined colander. Gather up the edges of the cheesecloth so you've got a ball of curds. Rinse under cold water for a minute or two, squeezing and moving the curds the whole time.

6. Squeeze the curds to get them as dry as possible, then transfer them into the dish you're going to use for storage.

7. Add the salt and heavy whipping cream and stir to incorporate, breaking the curds into smaller chunks as you go.

Nutrition per Serving
120 calories | 5g fat | 14g protein | 4g carbohydrate | 0g fiber |
4g net carbohydrate

Garlic and Onion Parmesan Crisps

Prep Time: 1 minute | *Cook Time:* 10 minutes |
Yield: About 33 crisps

1 cup grated Parmigiano-
Reggiano cheese

1 tablespoon onion powder

1 teaspoon garlic powder

½ teaspoon salt

½ teaspoon paprika

1. Add all ingredients into a mixing bowl and stir to combine.

2. Heat a heavy-bottomed pan over medium heat. Let it heat for 3 to 4 minutes before proceeding to step 3.

3. Place ½-tablespoon portions of your Parmesan mix directly on the hot pan. Let them cook until they just start to brown, about a minute and a half.

4. Using a spatula, remove each chip from the pan and place them on a paper towel.

5. Let cool before chomping.

Nutrition per 11 Crisps
115 calories | 7g fat | 10g protein | 1g carbohydrate | 0g fiber | 1g net carbohydrate

Main Dishes

Parmlette

The parmlette is a fantastic twist on the traditional egg omelet. It has a crispy Parmesan exterior and soft, creamy egg interior. You can fill it with anything you want but I've found the slight tartness of cherry tomatoes and smooth avocado is just the perfect combination.

Prep Time: 5 minutes | Cook Time: 12 to 15 minutes | Yield: 1 serving

1 tablespoon butter

2 tablespoons grated Parmigiano-Reggiano cheese

3 eggs

flesh of ½ avocado, sliced

2 cherry tomatoes, halved

3 big fresh basil leaves, julienned

1. Melt the butter in a large skillet over medium-low heat.

2. Evenly cover the bottom of the skillet with the Parmesan and cook for 3 to 5 minutes, until the Parmesan melts and just starts to brown.

3. In a bowl, scramble the eggs with a fork and pour them directly onto the Parmesan in the pan. Cook for about 3 minutes, until the eggs are set.

4. Add the avocado and tomatoes.

5. Fold the omelet and transfer to a plate.

6. Top with julienned basil and eat it that very second.

Nutrition per Serving

480 calories | 41g fat | 25g protein | 10g carbohydrate | 6g fiber | 4g net carbohydrate

Raspberry Fontina Hotcakes

Every once in a while you just want some darn pancakes. These are a low-carb, high-flavor variety of pancakes that will absolutely scratch that itch. They end up being really buttery and creamy and a tiny bit sweet and tart. You don't even need any type of syrup. Plus, being so high fat, they are very filling.

Prep Time: 5 minutes | Cook Time: 15 minutes | Yield: 3 (1-hotcake) servings

3 eggs

2 ounces cream cheese, softened

1 teaspoon vanilla extract

¾ cup almond flour

½ teaspoon baking powder

½ teaspoon salt

1½ cups shredded fontina cheese

¼ cup frozen raspberries

butter, for cooking

1. In a large mixing bowl, combine the eggs and cream cheese, and mix until smooth. Add vanilla extract.

2. Add the almond flour, baking powder, and salt, and mix again.

3. Add the fontina and raspberries, and mix a final time.

4. Melt about ½ tablespoon butter in a skillet over medium heat. Drop about ¾ cup batter onto the skillet and cook. When you see bubbles rise through the batter, it is about ready to flip, about 2 minutes on each side.

5. Add about ½ tablespoon butter before each hotcake and repeat until all the batter is gone. Serve hot.

Nutrition per Serving

460 calories | 39g fat | 23g protein | 5g carbohydrate | 1g fiber | 4g net carbohydrate

Raspberry Muffin Egg and Cheese Sandwich

I got this idea from a local cafe that would slice their homemade blueberry muffins in half and make breakfast sandwiches from them. Unfortunately that cafe closed, but its spirit lives on in this low-carb version of a berry breakfast sandwich. The nutmeg and raspberries in the muffin will provide a very nice contrast to the egg and cheese and hit that wonderful sweet-and-savory spot.

Prep Time: 2 minutes | **Cook Time:** 3 minutes | **Yield:** 1 serving

1 ounce cream cheese, softened

½ tablespoon butter, melted

3 tablespoons almond flour

½ teaspoon baking powder

¼ teaspoon salt

¼ teaspoon nutmeg

6 raspberries, frozen

1 egg, pan fried

1 slice cheddar cheese

1. Combine the softened cream cheese and melted butter in a small, high-walled microwave-safe dish and mix well. This dish will be the size of your muffin, so choose accordingly.

2. Add the almond flour, baking powder, salt, and nutmeg, and stir to combine.

3. Evenly space 3 raspberries in the dough. Microwave the mixture for 30 seconds.

4. Add the remaining 3 raspberries, also evenly spaced. The first three should have sunk to the bottom during the 30 seconds of microwaving.

5. Return to the microwave and cook for another 1½ minutes.

6. Using a towel, remove the dish from the microwave and immediately remove the muffin from the dish. The best way to get the muffin out of the dish is by tapping the inverted dish on a cutting board. Don't break it.

7. Once the muffin has cooled enough to handle, slice it in half, and put the fried egg and cheese in between the two slices.

Nutrition per Serving

464 calories | 41g fat | 20g protein | 8g carbohydrate | 3g fiber | 5g net carbohydrate

Caprese Hasselback Chicken

This caprese hasselback chicken is moist and flavorful when done. It evokes the freshness of a caprese salad but with more substance, because it is stuffed inside a chicken breast. Pair it with some broccoli or asparagus for a quick keto meal or enjoy with some rice or sweet potato for a low-carb meal.

Prep Time: 15 minutes | Cook Time: 20 minutes |
Yield: 4 servings

4 boneless skinless chicken breasts

3 tablespoons pesto

4 ounces fresh mozzarella, sliced into thin strips

3 tablespoons grated Parmigiano-Reggiano cheese

1 large plum tomato, sliced into thin strips

2 tablespoons olive oil

½ cup fresh basil, chopped

pinch sea salt

1. Preheat the oven to 400°F.

2. Slice each chicken breast 6 times crosswise, making sure not to slice all the way through.

3. Fill each slit in the chicken breasts with pesto, cheese, and tomato.

4. Place the stuffed chicken in an oiled baking dish with deep sides. Brush the chicken with olive oil.

5. Bake for 20 minutes.

6. Sprinkle salt and basil on top.

Nutrition per Serving
306 calories | 21g fat | 29g protein | 1g carbohydrate | 0g fiber | 1g net carbohydrate

Fontina and Sundried Tomato Stuffed Chicken Breast

This easy-to-make recipe still feels a bit fancy. Fontina cheese is excellent for melting but it can be pricey and may be difficult to find. Subbing fresh mozzarella or Swiss cheese works well.

Prep Time: 10 minutes | Cook Time: 25 minutes | Yield: 4 servings

4 boneless, skinless chicken breasts

2 tablespoons olive oil

1 teaspoon paprika

1 teaspoon garlic powder

½ teaspoon salt

1 teaspoon fresh ground black pepper

4 ounces fontina cheese

¼ cup sundried tomatoes

8 sprigs fresh thyme

1. Preheat the oven to 375°F.

2. Slice a pocket into each chicken breast.

3. In a small mixing bowl, combine the olive oil, paprika, garlic powder, salt, and pepper.

4. Using a brush, paint the exterior sides of chicken breasts with the oil and spice mixture.

5. Stuff 1 ounce fontina, a quarter of the sundried tomatoes, and 2 sprigs of thyme into each chicken breast.

6. Place the chicken breasts in a glass baking dish and bake for about 25 minutes.

Nutrition per Serving
317 calories | 17g fat | 34g protein | 5g carbohydrate | 1g fiber | 4g net carbohydrate

Crispy Spiced Chicken Tenders

I've seen many recipes for chicken tenders on the internet that claim to be "just like KFC," which I do not understand. Why would you want your homemade crispy chicken tenders to be just like a mediocre chain restaurant? These chicken tenders are, without a doubt, much better than KFC. The combination of spices and almond flour here makes for a nuanced and flavorful crunchy chicken tender, the likes of which you have not had before.

Prep Time: 10 minutes | Cook Time: 24 minutes | Yield: 4 servings

2 pounds boneless skinless chicken breast, sliced into 1½- to 2-inch-wide strips

2 eggs

1½ cups almond flour

½ tablespoon onion powder

½ tablespoon paprika

½ tablespoon garlic powder

½ tablespoon dried oregano

1 teaspoon ground salt

½ tablespoon fresh ground pepper

1 teaspoon cayenne pepper

1. Preheat the oven to 350°F.

2. Prepare your dredge stations. In one bowl, whisk the eggs. In a second bowl, combine the almond flour, onion powder, paprika, garlic powder, oregano, salt, pepper, and cayenne.

3. Dunk the chicken strips in the eggs, flip, and ensure the entire surface is coated.

4. Dredge the egg-coated chicken through the almond flour and spice mixture. Make sure the entire surface is coated.

5. Place a wire rack on a baking sheet and place the strips on the wire rack in a single layer. If you don't have a wire rack, you can place them directly on the baking sheet, but some of your coating may stick to the pan.

6. Bake for 12 minutes, flip, and bake for another 12 minutes.

7. Serve with your favorite low-carb dipping sauce.

Nutrition per Serving

430 calories | 23g fat | 38g protein | 6g carbohydrate | 4g fiber | 2g net carbohydrate

Flank Steak and Blue Cheese Salad

In my mind, there is nothing quite like the contrast of sharp blue cheese, fresh and cool lettuce, and warm, rich steak. This salad brings that all together for a fantastic medley of flavor and texture. I chose flank steak because it is generally thin and relatively inexpensive but does not skimp on flavor or tenderness. I don't recommend cooking the steak ahead of time with this recipe. Part of the magic is the heat from the steak partially melting some of your blue cheese crumbles.

Prep Time: 15 minutes | Cook Time: 2 minutes | Yield: 1 serving

2 cups chopped romaine lettuce hearts

¼ cup blue cheese crumbles

¼ medium red onion, sliced thin

½ avocado, cubed

¼ pound flank steak

2 tablespoons extra virgin olive oil

1. In a large bowl, combine the lettuce, blue cheese, onion, and avocado, and toss to combine.

2. Heat a medium-sized, heavy-bottomed skillet over medium heat for 5 minutes. Cook the steak for about a minute on each side for medium-rare. Slice it into thin strips and place the strips on top of the salad.

3. Drizzle with olive oil and eat immediately.

Nutrition per Serving
51 calories | 5g fat | 0.5g protein | 1g carbohydrate | 0.5g fiber | 0.5g net carbohydrate

Tuna Salad Zucchini Boats

I'm not sure why I have an obsession with stuffing vegetables full of delicious filling, but I do. These zucchini boats get bonus points for being handheld food, if that's your jam. They make a great quick lunch or dinner and can be served hot or cold. As written, the zucchini is raw and the tuna is cold, but if you want to turn it into a tuna melt, just add a half slice of Swiss cheese on the top and pop it in the oven for a bit. Try to use a mayonnaise that is not soy-oil based.

Prep Time: 15 minutes |
Yield: 4 servings

2 zucchini

2 cans tuna fish

½ cup mayonnaise

2 dill pickles, chopped

1 teaspoon celery salt

1 teaspoon fresh ground pepper

½ teaspoon salt

1 teaspoon garlic powder

1. Slice tops and bottoms off zucchini, slice lengthwise, and scoop out the seeds and some of the flesh with a spoon to make a stuffable trough.

2. In a mixing bowl, combine the tuna, mayo, pickles, celery salt, pepper, salt, and garlic powder. Mix thoroughly to combine.

3. Fill each zucchini with tuna salad.

Nutrition per Serving
290 calories | 21g fat | 17g protein | 4g carbohydrate | 1g fiber | 3g net carbohydrate

Ginger Bourbon Glazed Salmon

The astounding umami and nuance of the bourbon, balsamic, and ginger mixture in this recipe is mind blowing. Pair this with some broccoli or smashed cauliflower and you've got a truly stellar meal. Maybe drink some of the bourbon, too.

Prep Time: 5 minutes | *Cook Time:* 12 to 15 minutes | *Yield:* 3 (4-ounce) servings

3 (4-ounce) salmon fillets

1½ tablespoons ginger, minced

2 tablespoons soy sauce

4 tablespoons bourbon

3 tablespoons balsamic vinegar

2 tablespoons sesame oil

2 tablespoons sesame seeds

3 green onions, sliced

salted butter, for cooking

salt and pepper to taste

1. Preheat the oven to 450°F.

2. Melt the butter over medium heat in a heavy-bottomed skillet.

3. Add the ginger, soy sauce, bourbon, and balsamic vinegar to the skillet and bring to a simmer. Cook, stirring, until the mixture has reduced and become somewhat sticky.

4. Coat a baking sheet with the sesame oil and place salmon fillets skin-down on the pan. Brush them with sesame oil as well.

5. Bake the fillets for 5 minutes, remove from the oven, and sprinkle the sesame seeds on top, then return to oven for another 5 minutes.

6. Remove the salmon from the oven, pour the glaze over the fillets, and return to the oven for an additional 2 to 3 minutes. The salmon is done when it flakes easily with a fork.

7. Remove from the oven, garnish with green onions, season with salt and pepper, and serve immediately.

Nutrition per Serving

334 calories | 13g fat | 22g protein | 12g carbohydrate | 2g fiber | 10g net carbohydrate

Buffalo Chicken Stuffed Poblano Peppers

While traditional stuffed poblano peppers do not have any buffalo chicken dip inside them, I find this combination of the spicy and creamy chicken dip with the mild pepper to be divine. Pair one of these peppers with a couple of fried eggs or use it as a salad topper. However you choose to consume the finished product, this is a quick and easy flavor explosion.

Prep Time: 25 minutes | *Cook Time:* 20 minutes |
Yield: 4 servings

4 medium poblano peppers

1 recipe Buffalo Chicken Dip (page 177)

¼ medium red onion, diced

½ cup fresh cilantro

olive oil, for cooking

1. Preheat the oven to 400°F.

2. Coat a baking sheet with the oil.

3. Slice the tops off the peppers, make one lengthwise slice down the side, split the peppers, and remove the seeds.

4. Stuff each pepper to the gills with buffalo chicken dip and place them in a single layer on the baking sheet.

5. Bake for 20 minutes until the peppers are soft and charred in a few spots.

6. Sprinkle onion and cilantro on top right before serving.

Nutrition per Serving
415 calories | 31g fat | 22g protein | 12g carbohydrate | 4g fiber | 8g net carbohydrate

Peanut Chicken Kabobs

Prep Time: 10 minutes | Cook Time: 30 minutes |
Yield: 4 servings

For the sauce

½ cup no-sugar-added peanut butter

2 tablespoons soy sauce

1 tablespoon hot sauce (preferably Valentina)

¼ cup broth or water

1 teaspoon garlic powder

1 teaspoon ginger powder

For the kabobs

wooden or metal skewers

4 boneless, skinless chicken breasts

2 bell peppers

1 red onion

1 (8-ounce) package button mushrooms

1. If using wooden skewers, soak in water overnight to prevent them catching on fire in the oven.

2. Preheat the oven to 450°F.

3. Combine all the sauce ingredients in a blender or food processor and blend until smooth. Transfer to a large bowl.

4. Chop the chicken, bell peppers, and onion into 1-inch sections.

5. Place chopped chicken in the bowl of peanut sauce and toss to coat.

6. Thread the skewers with alternating pieces of sauce-coated chicken and vegetables. Pack the skewers tightly.

7. Place the skewers on a lipped baking pan. Bake for 25 to 30 minutes, flipping once.

Nutrition per Serving

448 calories | 20g fat | 52g protein | 16g carbohydrate | 6g fiber | 10g net carbohydrate

Deconstructed Philly Cheese Steak

I've never actually eaten a true Philly cheese steak sandwich, so I was really just guessing at the authenticity of flavor. If you are a diehard Philly cheese steak fan and don't think this approximates what you love, scratch out the title and call it "Robert's Steak and Pepper Delight." It'll still be delicious.

Prep Time: 10 minutes | Cook Time: 15 to 20 minutes | Yield: 2 servings

¾ pound ribeye steak

½ medium red onion, sliced thin

2 green bell peppers, sliced into 2-inch-wide spears

1 cup shredded mozzarella cheese

4 ounces cream cheese, softened

butter, for cooking

salt and pepper to taste

1. Preheat the oven to 350°F.

2. Melt the butter over medium heat in a heavy-bottomed frying pan. Allow the pan to get *really* hot, then sear the steak on each side for no more than a minute. Remove from the pan and set aside to cool.

3. In the same pan, sauté the onions until they are limp and translucent, about 5 minutes.

4. Lay the peppers flat, inside up, on a baking sheet.

5. Slice the steak into very thin strips.

6. In a mixing bowl, combine the mozzarella cheese, cream cheese, onions, steak strips, and salt and pepper. Mix well.

7. Spoon your steak and cheese mixture onto the green pepper spears.

8. Bake for 10 to 15 minutes depending on how you like your steak cooked.

Nutrition per Serving
530 calories | 42g fat | 26g protein | 18g carbohydrate | 6g fiber | 12g net carbohydrate

Ginger Beef Dumplings

I adapted this and the following recipe from two sources: I got the basic idea for the fillings from some dumplings my wife and I used to make on the regular, and I got the cabbage shell idea from a truly amazing individual in the keto space who publishes recipes under the name Headbanger's Kitchen. Look him up on YouTube. You're welcome.

Prep Time: 15 minutes | Cook Time: 25 minutes |
Yield: 4 servings

7 to 10 cabbage leaves

½ pound ground beef

1 teaspoon soy sauce, plus more to serve

1 teaspoon rice wine vinegar

½ tablespoon fresh ginger, minced

½ tablespoon garlic, minced

½ teaspoon ground cayenne pepper

pinch ground cloves

2 tablespoons sesame oil

sriracha, to serve

1. In a large pot, boil the cabbage leaves for about 5 minutes, remove, and let cool.

2. While leaves are cooling, combine the ground beef, soy sauce, rice wine vinegar, ginger, garlic, cayenne, and cloves in a bowl, and mix well.

3. Slice each cabbage leaf in half.

4. Stuff each cabbage leaf half with filling and fold them over to close. Aim for fat dumplings that can still be closed.

5. In a lightly oiled stove-top steamer, cook the dumplings over a simmer for 15 minutes to mostly cook the beef, further soften the cabbage, and seal the dumplings.

6. Heat the sesame oil in a skillet and fry the dumplings on each side until browned, about 2 minutes per side.

7. Serve with soy sauce and sriracha.

Nutrition per Serving
240 calories | 17g fat | 17g protein | 5g carbohydrate | 2g fiber | 3g net carbohydrate

Spinach and Cream Cheese Dumplings

Prep Time: 15 minutes | Cook Time: 10 minutes |
Yield: 4 servings

7 to 10 cabbage leaves

4 cups fresh spinach

4 ounces cream
cheese, softened

2 tablespoons sesame oil

soy sauce and
sriracha, to serve

1. In a large pot, boil the cabbage leaves for about 5 minutes, remove, and let cool.

2. While leaves are cooling, sauté the spinach over medium heat until thoroughly wilted. Remove from heat and let cool.

3. Slice each cabbage leaf in half.

4. Squeeze the spinach to remove as much liquid as you possibly can.

5. Combine the spinach and cream cheese in a mixing bowl and mix until well combined.

6. Stuff each cabbage leaf half with filling and fold them over to close. Aim for fat dumplings that can still be closed.

7. In a lightly oiled stove-top steamer, cook the dumplings over a simmer for 2 to 3 minutes to further soften the cabbage and seal the dumplings.

8. Heat the sesame oil in a skillet and fry the dumplings on each side until browned, about 2 minutes per side.

9. Serve with soy sauce and sriracha.

Nutrition per Serving

*240 calories | 22g fat | 4g protein | 7g carbohydrate | 2g fiber |
5g net carbohydrate*

Slow Cooker Beef Stew

If your beef stew is not hearty, forget about it. This beef stew is very, very hearty. I recommend prepping your ingredients the night before, throwing everything in the slow cooker before you go out in the morning, and then being greeted by the nourishing aroma of beef stew as soon as you get home. It is unbeatable in the winter. If you want it for the ketogenic portion of the diet, skip the potatoes and carrots and sub another cup of beef broth for the red wine.

Prep Time: 25 minutes | *Cook Time:* 6 to 10 hours |
Yield: 8 servings

4 tablespoons olive oil

2 pounds trimmed beef chuck, cut into 1- to 2-inch cubes

1 medium onion, chopped

1 cup beef broth, divided

2 teaspoons garlic, minced

5 red potatoes, diced

3 medium carrots, sliced

4 medium celery stalks, sliced

1 cup of red cooking wine

1 (14.5-ounce) can diced tomatoes, drained

2 bay leaves

2 sprigs fresh thyme or 1 teaspoon dried thyme

1 teaspoon dried rosemary

1 teaspoon dried oregano

1 teaspoon dried parsley

½ teaspoon allspice

8 ounces mushrooms, sliced

salt and pepper to taste

1. Heat the olive oil in a heavy-bottomed skillet until shimmering. Sear the beef on all sides, remove from skillet, and set aside.

2. Add the onions to the skillet and cook until translucent, about 5 minutes.

3. Pour 1 to 2 tablespoons of broth into the skillet, stir, and scrape the bottom of the skillet with a wooden spoon to dislodge all the flavorful brown bits.

4. Add the beef, onions, remaining beef broth, and all other ingredients to a slow cooker.

5. Cook on low for 9 to 10 hours, medium 7 to 8 hours, or high 6 to 7 hours, removing the lid for the last hour or two to allow some reduction and thickening. Stir occasionally.

6. Remove the bay leaves before serving.

Nutrition per Serving

438 calories | 26g fat | 24g protein | 23g carbohydrate | 3g fiber | 20g net carbohydrate

Sausage and Rosemary Stuffed Acorn Squash

If you've never had acorn squash before, you're in for a treat. It is slightly sweet but not quite as sweet as a butternut squash. The flesh of the squash is hearty and tender. Combined with the sausage and rosemary, it makes for a very filling, very flavorful meal. This recipe will not work well for the strict ketosis portion of the diet. You could replace the squash with zucchini or green bell pepper and make it work.

Prep Time: 15 minutes | Cook Time: 1 hour 15 minutes | Yield: 4 servings

2 acorn squash

2 tablespoons olive oil

1 teaspoon ground cumin

1 pound ground sausage of choice

½ medium red onion, chopped

2 stalks celery, chopped

2 tablespoons fresh rosemary, chopped

1 cup shredded Parmigiano-Reggiano cheese, divided

salt and pepper to taste

1. Preheat the oven to 400°F.

2. Slice the ends off the acorn squash, and then slice each in half. Spoon out the seeds and discard.

3. Brush the inside of each squash with olive oil and sprinkle with salt, pepper, and cumin.

4. Bake the squash for 40 minutes to an hour. When you can easily pierce the flesh with a fork, it is done.

5. While the squash is baking, sauté the sausage over medium heat in a skillet for about 5 minutes, then remove the sausage from the pan.

6. In the same pan, sauté the onion and celery for roughly 2 minutes.

7. In a medium mixing bowl, combine the sausage, celery, onion, rosemary, and ¾ cup cheese, and mix to combine.

8. Once the squash is finished baking, remove it from the oven, fill each half with sausage mixture, and return it to the oven for another 15 minutes.

9. Remove the squash from the oven, sprinkle with remaining cheese, and serve.

Nutrition per Serving

550 calories | 41g fat | 24g protein | 24g carbohydrate | 4g fiber | 20g net carbohydrate

Butternut Squash, Sage, and Apple Soup

The combination of butternut and apple is a no-brainer for soup but the added oomph of sage takes it to another level. This soup is sweet and savory at the same time and all autumn. It is basically fall in a bowl. If ya feelin fancy, swirl in another spoonful of coconut milk and sprinkle a few pumpkin seeds on top right before serving.

This recipe is mostly carbohydrate and that's okay. It is not intended for the full ketogenic portion of the diet.

Prep Time: 20 minutes | Cook Time: 45 minutes | Yield: 6 servings

1 tablespoon olive oil

1 tablespoon diced fresh garlic

½ medium yellow onion, diced

2 cups vegetable stock

3 to 4 pounds butternut squash, seeded, peeled, and chopped

½ carrot, chopped

1 Granny Smith apple, cored and chopped

½ teaspoon salt

½ teaspoon fresh ground black pepper

½ teaspoon ground nutmeg

pinch cayenne pepper

2 teaspoons ground sage

½ cup unsweetened coconut milk

1. In a medium pot heat the oil over medium heat. Sauté the garlic for about a minute then add the onion and sauté until the onions turn translucent, about 5 minutes.

2. Add the vegetable stock, butternut squash, and carrot. Bring to a boil, then reduce to a simmer. Cover and cook for 30 minutes.

3. Add the apple, cover, and cook for another 10 minutes.

4. Blend the soup until it is smooth. You can either use an immersion blender in the pot or transfer to a regular blender in batches. Either way, don't burn yourself.

5. Add the salt, pepper, nutmeg, cayenne, and sage. Cook for 10 more minutes.

6. Stir in the coconut milk. Serve hot or cooled.

Nutrition per Serving
175 calories | 4g fat | 3g protein | 38g carbohydrate | 7g fiber | 31g net carbohydrate

Sweet Potato Curry

I love a good curry anything. And the beauty of a curry is that there is no set recipe or definition of what a curry should be. It really just means something like stir-fry. Of course, there are some spices we associate with a good curry, and I've included those here. This dish is vegetarian by design but if you'd like, you can always add a protein of choice. Obviously, being sweet potato-based, this recipe is intended for the second portion of the diet. If you think it sounds good and can't wait to get to the second phase to try it, sub paneer, tofu, or chicken for the sweet potato and change the cook time accordingly.

Prep Time: 15 minutes | *Cook Time:* 30 minutes |
Yield: 2 servings

2 tablespoons butter

1 can unsweetened coconut milk

1 tablespoon red curry paste

1 teaspoon cumin

1 teaspoon turmeric

½ teaspoon salt

1 large sweet potato, cubed

½ cup cashews

1 green bell pepper, seeded and chopped

8 ounces cremini mushrooms, chopped

½ medium red onion, roughly chopped

riced cauliflower, to serve

½ cup fresh cilantro, chopped fine

1. Melt butter in heavy-bottomed skillet over medium heat.

2. Add the coconut milk, curry paste, cumin, turmeric, and salt, and stir to combine. Bring to a simmer.

3. Add the sweet potato, cover, and cook for 20 minutes, stirring occasionally.

4. Add the cashews, bell pepper, mushrooms, and onion and cook uncovered for another 10 minutes.

5. Serve over riced cauliflower with fresh cilantro sprinkled on top.

Nutrition per Serving

437 calories | 30g fat | 12g protein | 36g carbohydrate | 8g fiber | 28g net carbohydrate

Side Dishes

Herbed Mashed Cauliflower

Some people require mashed potatoes to live. I am not one of those people, but my wife is. When I started eating a low-carbohydrate diet, I skipped out on the potatoes most of the time, so I decided to come up with a low-carb version of mashed potatoes. Cauliflower has a mild enough taste that it can be made to taste almost exactly like fancy mashed potatoes—you know, the kind with herbs.

Prep Time: 15 minutes | *Cook Time:* 20 minutes |
Yield: 4 servings

1 medium head cauliflower

4 ounces cream cheese

¼ cup sour cream

2 tablespoons butter, plus more to serve

2 teaspoons dried oregano

2 teaspoons dried thyme

2 teaspoons garlic, minced

1 teaspoon salt

1 teaspoon fresh ground black pepper

1. Trim the cauliflower and break into florets. Chop up the stem into ½-inch chunks.

2. Steam the cauliflower using a stove-top steamer or in a microwave until soft and tender, about 10 minutes with heavy steam or 15 minutes in the microwave.

3. Using a kitchen towel, squeeze as much of the liquid out of the cauliflower as you can. Careful—the liquid will be hot.

4. Place the cauliflower, cream cheese, sour cream, butter, oregano, thyme, garlic, salt, and pepper into a blender or food processor and blend until it is the smoothness you desire. If you like your mashed potato chunky, leave out some of the stem pieces and add them in after you've blended the rest smooth.

5. Serve immediately while still hot, with an additional pat of butter on top.

Nutrition per Serving

225 calories | 19g fat | 5g protein | 11g carbohydrate | 4g fiber | 7g net carbohydrate

Sesame Zucchini Rounds

One of the great things about a ketogenic diet is getting to absolutely coat your vegetables in delicious fat. Whether you use butter, cheese, or a flavorful oil like sesame oil, it makes getting your fiber and phytonutrients much more enjoyable.

Prep Time: 5 minutes | Cook Time: 3 minutes | Yield: 2 servings

1 tablespoon sesame oil

1 tablespoon sesame seeds

1 zucchini, sliced into ¼-inch-thick rounds

pinch sea salt

1. Heat oil and sesame seeds over medium heat in a frying pan.

2. Sauté the zucchini rounds in the oil and seeds for about 3 minutes, tossing to coat. They are done with they just start to soften. You want to have some crunch left.

3. Remove from heat, add salt to taste, and serve immediately.

Nutrition per Serving
100 calories | 9g fat | 1g protein | 4g carbohydrate | 2g fiber | 2g net carbohydrate

Sage-Roasted Broccoli

Broccoli is one of my favorite vegetables and I love to highlight its natural flavors. I think sage is an underutilized spice. Before I started cooking more, I'd only encountered it in breakfast sausage, and I didn't even know that's what I was tasting. The combination of sage and chili powder makes for a rich, earthy side that pairs very well with Caprese Hasselback Chicken (page 146) or Ginger Bourbon Glazed Salmon (page 152).

Prep Time: 5 minutes | Cook Time: 20 minutes | Yield: 5 servings

1 pound fresh broccoli, cut into florets

4 tablespoons olive oil, divided

2 tablespoons ground sage

2 teaspoons chili powder

2 teaspoons salt

1. Preheat the oven to 425°F.

2. In a large mixing bowl, toss the broccoli in 3 tablespoons olive oil.

3. Sprinkle the sage, chili powder, and salt over the broccoli, then toss to coat.

4. Place the broccoli in a single layer on a metal baking sheet. Bake for 10 minutes, flip, and bake for another 10 minutes.

5. Serve drizzled with the remaining oil.

Nutrition per Serving
131 calories | 11g fat | 3g protein | 7g carbohydrate | 3g fiber | 4g net carbohydrate

Roasted Cabbage

Cabbage is one of those vegetables that is woefully underutilized in the American diet. It is all too often relegated to the world of coleslaw and the occasional sauerkraut on top of a hot dog. No more! This roasted cabbage recipe puts this brassica family member (the same family as broccoli, brussels sprouts, and cauliflower) in the front and center. The blackening and caramelization that will occur on the outer leaves provides a fantastic contrast to the tender and mild inner portion.

Prep Time: 5 minutes | Cook Time: 20 minutes |
Yield: 8 servings

1 medium head cabbage

3 tablespoons avocado oil

coarse sea salt

fresh ground black pepper

1. Preheat the oven to 500°F.

2. Slice the cabbage into 8 thick wedges.

3. Place the wedges on a metal baking pan in a single layer. Drizzle them with oil and liberally sprinkle with salt and pepper, then flip the wedges to drizzle and sprinkle the other side.

4. Roast the cabbage for 10 minutes on each side. They should be deeply browned with some blackened spots.

Nutrition per Serving
51 calories | 5g fat | 0.5g protein | 1g carbohydrate | 0.5g fiber | 0.5g net carbohydrate

Note: If you don't have avocado oil, use extra virgin olive oil, reduce the heat to 400°F, and increase the cooking time by 3 to 5 minutes per side. Avocado oil is one of the only oils stable at 500°F, but it can be difficult to find or prohibitively expensive.

Turnips Au Gratin

Turnips, by their nature, are bitter. If you forget their birthday *even once,* they will never let you forget it. It is this bitterness that necessitates the seemingly unreasonable cook time. This long, low cooking mellows out the turnips quite a lot, and they become very mild and pleasant. Don't skip the super-long cook time.

Prep Time: 15 minutes | Cook Time: 2½ hours |
Yield: 6 servings

2 large turnips, trimmed, peeled, and sliced paper thin

8 ounces cheddar cheese, shredded

1 cup grated Parmigiano-Reggiano cheese

3 tablespoons butter, in thin slices

1 tablespoon dried oregano

1 tablespoon garlic powder

1 tablespoon onion powder

1 teaspoon salt

1 teaspoon fresh ground black pepper

1. Preheat the oven to 250°F.

2. Place the turnips in a slightly overlapping layer on the bottom of a deep baking dish. Then top with the cheddar, Parmigiano-Reggiano, butter, oregano, garlic, onion, salt, and pepper, in that order. Add a second layer of turnips and the remaining ingredients. Try to use roughly an even amount of ingredients for each layer and try to finish with a layer of cheddar cheese.

3. Place your cheesy turnip stack in the oven, covered in foil, and bake for 2 hours. Remove foil and bake for another half hour.

Nutrition per Serving
245 calories | 20g fat | 11g protein | 7g carbohydrate | 2g fiber | 5g net carbohydrate

Baked Okra

Prep Time: 15 minutes | *Cook Time:* 30 minutes |
Yield: 2 servings

2 tablespoons olive oil

2 teaspoons cumin

1 teaspoon salt

1 teaspoon fresh ground black pepper

½ pound okra, washed and thoroughly dried

1. Preheat the oven to 400°F.

2. In a large bowl, combine the olive oil, cumin, salt, and pepper.

3. Toss the okra in the spiced oil mixture and arrange in a single row on a metal baking sheet.

4. Bake for 15 minutes, flip, and bake for another 15 minutes, or until soft.

5. Remove from the oven. Let cool for about 3 minutes, then serve with your favorite low-carb dipping sauce.

Nutrition per Serving
170 calories | 14g fat | 3g protein | 10g carbohydrate | 4g fiber | 6g net carbohydrate

Buffalo Chicken Dip

Creamy and pleasantly spicy, this dip is a versatile side to be served with Tortilla Chips (page 128) or used as an ingredient in Buffalo Chicken Stuffed Poblano Peppers (page 154). It comes together quickly and is great hot or cold. A vinegar-based hot sauce like Texas Pete is my favorite to use for this recipe.

Prep Time: 5 minutes | Cook Time: 25 minutes | Yield: 6 servings

8 ounces cream cheese, softened

1 cup shredded cooked chicken breast

½ cup red hot sauce of choice

¼ cup low-carb blue cheese dressing

1 cup shredded Colby-Monterey Jack cheese blend

½ teaspoon salt

½ teaspoon black pepper

1. Preheat the oven to 350°F.

2. Combine all ingredients in a mixing bowl and stir until combined.

3. Transfer the dip to a shallow ceramic dish and bake for 25 minutes. If you want the top to be gooey, cover with tin foil. If you want the top to be browned and a little crispy, bake uncovered.

Nutrition per Serving
345 calories | 29g fat | 17g protein | 3g carbohydrate | 0g fiber | 3g net carbohydrate

Spicy Collard Greens

In the Southern United States, collard greens are a big deal. You see them cooked with pork fat, in vinegar, with hot sauce, and as a New Year's Day tradition with black eyed peas called beans 'n greens. Collard greens are also amazingly nutritious and a great vehicle for olive oil. My variation on spicy collard greens lets them simmer in their own flavorful juices, leading to the incredible sensation of biting into juicy, smoky, spicy greens. Use your favorite smoky hot sauce for this recipe.

Prep Time: 15 minutes | Cook Time: 30 to 40 minutes | Yield: 4 servings

2 large bunches collard greens

1 tablespoon olive oil

2 slices thick bacon or pork belly, diced

1 teaspoon garlic, minced

½ red onion, chopped

1 fresh jalapeno pepper, seeded and chopped

8 ounces cremini mushrooms, chopped

½ cup beef stock

1 tablespoon soy sauce

1 tablespoon hot sauce of choice

2 teaspoons fresh ground black pepper

1. Wash and chop the greens. Fold the leaves in half and in half again. Slice them horizontally into strips about 2 inches wide. Trim the bit of the stem that does not have any leaf growth.

2. Heat the oil in a large pot over medium heat and toss in the bacon or pork belly. Cook 3 to 5 minutes, then add in the garlic, onion, and jalapeno, and sauté for another 3 minutes.

3. Add the mushrooms and sauté until they soften and release their liquid, about 5 minutes.

4. Add the collard greens and stir well to get the flavors all mixed up. Cook for about a minute.

5. Add the beef stock, soy sauce, hot sauce, and black pepper. Cover, bring to a simmer, and cook for 20 to 25 minutes, stirring occasionally.

6. Use tongs or a slotted spoon to serve.

Nutrition per Serving

110 calories | 6g fat | 7g protein | 7g carbohydrate | 5g fiber | 2g net carbohydrate

Note: The best way to wash any type of green leafy vegetable is to fill a basin (sinks work well) with cold water and put the whole batch of greens in. Swish them around a good bit, drain the basin, and repeat the process of filling and swishing. This should allow any dirt, sand, or whatever else is trapped in the leaves to sink to the bottom of the basin while the greens float.

Desserts

Coconut Avocado Fiesta Pops

If you've never had avocado in a dessert before, get ready. The creamy, silky goodness is just amazing. Combined with coconut, lime, and tequila, it makes for a perfect treat on a hot day. If you want a perfectly smooth pop, you can omit the shredded coconut. I like the bit of texture.

Prep Time: 5 minutes, plus chill time |
Yield: 6 servings

1 avocado, scooped

1 (13.5-ounce) can coconut milk

3 tablespoons tequila

2 tablespoons lime juice

¼ cup fresh mint leaves

2 tablespoons unsweetened shredded coconut

1. Place the avocado flesh, coconut milk, tequila, lime juice, and mint leaves in blender, and blend until smooth.

2. Add the shredded coconut and pulse to combine.

3. Pour mixture into ice pop molds and freeze overnight.

Nutrition per Serving
171 calories | 14g fat | 1g protein | 6g carbohydrate | 5.5g fiber | 0.5g net carbohydrate

Lemon Zest Yogurt Cake

This is a low-carb variation on a traditional French dessert bread recipe. It is moist and somewhat sweet with a little bit of tang. It does not rise very much in the oven, so don't worry about that. It goes really well with fancy tea time, if one is so inclined to participate in fancy tea time.

Prep Time: 5 minutes | Cook Time: 50 to 55 minutes | Yield: 8 servings

1½ cups almond flour

½ cup coconut flour

1 teaspoon baking powder

½ teaspoon salt

¾ cup Greek yogurt

2 eggs

1 teaspoon vanilla extract

1 lemon, zested

butter, for greasing

1. Preheat the oven to 350°F and thoroughly grease a loaf pan with butter.

2. Sift the almond flour, coconut flour, baking powder, and salt into a medium mixing bowl. Then add the Greek yogurt, eggs, vanilla extract, and lemon zest, and stir until well combined.

3. Pour the batter into the loaf pan and bake for 50 to 55 minutes, or until toothpick or fork tines can be inserted and removed cleanly.

4. Let cool for 15 minutes before cutting.

Nutrition per Serving
146 calories | 10g fat | 8g protein | 7g carbohydrate | 4g fiber | 3g net carbohydrate

Cheesecake

Cheesecake doesn't need much work to be converted to a low-carb dessert since it is mostly cheese already. Whip up a low-carb crust and you're good to go. This version comes out dense and creamy and a little less sweet than traditional cheesecake. I think it is an improvement, but if you prefer very sweet cheesecake, add ¼ cup erythritol.

Prep Time: 20 minutes | Cook Time: 45 to 50 minutes, plus rest time | Yield: 10 servings

for crust

½ cup almond flour

½ cup coconut flour

¼ cup shredded coconut

½ cup melted butter

½ teaspoon cinnamon

½ teaspoon nutmeg

for filling

16 ounces cream cheese, softened

¾ cup sour cream

3 eggs

1 teaspoon vanilla extract

1 teaspoon lemon zest

1. Combine all the crust ingredients in a bowl and mix well.

2. Line the bottom of a cake tin or deep-walled circular glass baking dish with the crust mixture. Press it with your hands to make sure it is of an even depth all around. Place the dish in the fridge while preparing the filling.

3. Preheat the oven to 320°F.

4. Combine all of the filling ingredients in a bowl and mix until smooth and well combined. This is easiest with a hand or stand mixer, but a whisk and a lot of work will get it done.

5. Pour the filling into the crust. Give it a little shake or tap on the counter to make sure it settles evenly.

6. Place the cheesecake in the oven, along with about a cup of water in an oven-safe dish.

7. Bake for 45 to 50 minutes, or until toothpick or fork tines can be inserted and removed cleanly.

8. Turn off the oven and open the door, but do not remove the cake for another 30 minutes.

9. Remove the cake and place it in the fridge for at least an hour but preferably overnight.

Nutrition per Serving
322 calories | 31g fat | 6g protein | 7g carbohydrate | 3g fiber | 4g net carbohydrate

Strawberry Cream Gummies

I was baffled when I learned how easy it is to make gummies. This is a simple recipe but the variations are endless if the texture is something you enjoy.

Prep Time: 15 minutes, plus rest time |
Yield: 6 (4-gummy) servings

2 (0.25-ounce) packets unflavored gelatin

½ cup cool water

½ cup heavy whipping cream

½ cup fresh strawberries, pureed

1. Sprinkle the gelatin on top of the cool water and let bloom for at least 5 minutes.

2. Heat the heavy whipping cream in a saucepan over medium heat until steaming, about 5 minutes. Do not let it boil.

3. Remove the cream from the heat, stir in the strawberry puree, and mix well.

4. Combine the gelatin and cream mixtures and transfer to 24-cavity candy mold.

5. Refrigerate for at least an hour.

Nutrition per Serving
80 calories | 8g fat | 2g protein | 0.5g carbohydrate | 0g fiber | 0.5g net carbohydrate

Blueberry Chia Pudding

Chia seeds are an often-overlooked nutrient powerhouse. They are packed with fiber and fat, which is a rare combination (I'm looking at you, avocados), and they have the strange ability to form a gel. This can be useful in a variety of cooking applications, not least of which is making a healthy pudding. I used almond milk in the recipe, but you can use any type of liquid you want.

Prep Time: 1 minute, plus rest time |
Yield: 4 servings

¾ cup blueberries

1½ cups unsweetened almond milk

½ cup chia seeds

1 teaspoon vanilla extract

½ teaspoon cinnamon

½ teaspoon cardamom

1. In a medium bowl, mash the blueberries with a fork until you have a blueberry paste.

2. Add all other ingredients and mix until well combined.

3. Cover and refrigerate for a minimum of 6 hours.

Nutrition per Serving
157 calories | 7g fat | 7g protein | 18g carbohydrate | 13g fiber | 5g net carbohydrate

Drinks

Citrus Electrolyte Refresher—Electroaide

You need to replenish your electrolytes while you are in ketosis or if you are participating in heavily taxing activities that make you sweat a lot. This drink is a fantastic and refreshing way to get those vital nutrients. I don't usually use difficult-to-obtain ingredients, but the vitamin C powder gives this drink an extra kick that is worth it if you can find it. Unfortunately, the internet is your best bet for locating vitamin C powder. It may also be listed as ascorbic acid powder. That's just a different name for vitamin C. Potassium salt is easy to find, though you may not have known that's what it was when you saw it. Table salt alternatives sold in grocery stores are almost all potassium salts. They will be with the regular salt in the store. Common brands are NoSalt and Nu-Salt.

Prep Time: 5 minutes | *Cook Time:* 1 minute | *Yield:* 4 servings

32 ounces warm water

½ tablespoon lemon or lime juice

2 teaspoons salt

1 teaspoon potassium salt

4 teaspoons vitamin C powder

Combine all ingredients in pitcher of adequate size and mix to combine. Store in the refrigerator until ready to serve.

Nutrition per Serving
0 calories | 0g fat | 0g protein | 0g carbohydrate | 0g fiber | 0g net carbohydrate

Peanut Butter and Jelly Protein Smoothie

This smoothie is perfect for a quick breakfast or snack. It has the same rich consistency as traditional smoothies but is not a sugar bomb like most banana-based smoothies. The flavor hearkens to a good ole PB & J sandwich.

Prep Time: 5 minutes |
Yield: 1 smoothie

½ cup silken tofu

½ cup frozen strawberries

2 tablespoons no-sugar-added peanut butter

1 cup no-sugar-added almond milk

1 scoop MCT oil powder or low-carb protein powder of choice

Combine all ingredients in a blender. Blend until smooth.

Nutrition Info per Smoothie

345 kcal | 13g protein | 27g fat | 12g carbohydrate | 6g fiber | 6g net carbohydrate

Dressings and Sauces

Butter

Making your own butter is surprisingly easy. If you have a stand mixer, hand mixer, or food processor, making butter is easy-peasy.

Prep Time: 1 minute | Cook Time: 15 minutes | Yield: 16 (1-tablespoon) servings

3 cups heavy whipping cream

¼ cup very cold water

salt to taste

1. Pour heavy whipping cream into a medium bowl or the work bowl of stand mixer or food processor.

2. Mix on high until you get solid separation, about 5 minutes. You should have some clear fluid and some thicker chunks of cream.

3. Add the water and mix for another 2 to 3 minutes.

4. Pour the butter and milk liquid into a colander. Using your hands, squeeze all the liquid you possibly can out of your butter.

5. Transfer to the container you want to store it in, add salt to taste, and mix to combine.

Nutrition per Tablespoon
100 calories | 12g fat | 0g protein | 0g carbohydrate | 0g fiber | 0g net carbohydrate

Cilantro Lime Chili Butter

Spiced butter is a simple way to make something already great even better. This recipe is refreshing with the slightest little kick. You can make a batch ahead of time and instantly add an explosion of flavor to anything you want. I personally love it melted on a mild fish like cod or used to spice up a vegetable like cabbage or cauliflower. If you are one of the genetically unfortunate individuals to whom cilantro tastes like soap, sub green onions.

Prep Time: 1 minute | Cook Time: 12 to 15 minutes | Yield: 12 (1-tablespoon) servings

2 sticks salted butter, room temperature

¼ cup fresh cilantro, chopped fine

1 tablespoon lime juice

½ teaspoon chili powder

pinch cayenne pepper

1. Place the butter in a medium bowl and whisk until creamed. Use a hand or stand mixer if you can.

2. Add the rest of the ingredients and whisk until combined.

3. Place in airtight container and refrigerate until needed.

Nutrition per Serving
134 calories | 15g fat | 0g protein | 0g carbohydrate | 0g fiber | 0g net carbohydrate

Magic Olive Oil and Vinegar Dressing

I call this dressing "magic" because vinegar has consistently been shown to reduce blood glucose spikes following a meal. So really, this is just tasty dressing that will help your body better handle the carbohydrates in whatever you put this dressing on. It is tangy and flavorful and I find it pairs well with salads that include some creamy cheese, like goat cheese.

Prep Time: 5 minutes |
Yield: 16 (1-ounce) servings

1 cup extra virgin olive oil

½ cup apple cider vinegar

1 teaspoon dried oregano

1 teaspoon dried thyme

1 teaspoon ground black pepper

1 teaspoon dried rosemary

1 teaspoon crushed red pepper flakes

Mix all ingredients in the container you want to store your dressing in. If kept cool and away from light, this dressing can be stored for up to 3 months.

Nutrition per Serving
120 calories | 14g fat | 0g protein | 0g carbohydrate | 0g fiber | 0g net carbohydrate

Creamy Cheese Sauce

I don't even have to describe this, do I? It is cheese sauce. It goes on everything.

Prep Time: 5 minutes | *Cook Time:* 12 to 15 minutes | *Yield:* 6 (3-tablespoon) servings

2 tablespoons butter

¾ cup heavy whipping cream

2 tablespoons cream cheese

5 ounces sharp cheddar cheese, grated

½ teaspoon paprika

salt and pepper to taste

1. Melt the butter in a saucepan over medium-low heat.

2. Add the heavy whipping cream and continue to heat until it is simmering. Do not let it boil.

3. Add the cream cheese, stirring until it is totally combined.

4. Add the cheddar cheese in batches, stirring continuously. As some melts, add more until it is all incorporated.

5. Add the paprika, taste, and add salt and pepper to taste.

Nutrition per Serving

250 calories | 24g fat | 7g protein | 1g carbohydrate | 0g fiber | 1g net carbohydrate

Bolognese

This traditional Italian meat sauce is pronounced *bo-lo-naise*. It is great over vegetable noodles or as a filling for zucchini boats. It takes a long time to make but it makes a lot and is worth the trouble. It is rich and filing in the way that only slow-made meat sauces can be.

Prep Time: 20 minutes | Cook Time: 4 hours 15 minutes | Yield: 24 (2-tablespoon) servings

2 tablespoons butter

1 tablespoon olive oil

1 large onion, chopped small

3 pounds ground beef

8 ounces pancetta, chopped small

2 stalks celery, chopped small

1 large carrot, chopped small

6 cloves garlic, minced

1 cup red wine

1 (28-ounce) can no-sugar-added tomato puree

1 cup heavy whipping cream

2 cups beef stock

salt and pepper to taste

1. Melt the butter and heat the olive oil in a large, heavy-bottomed pot over medium heat.

2. Add the onion, beef, and pancetta, and cook until the meat is browned and the onion is translucent, 6 to 8 minutes, stirring to break up the beef into small pieces.

3. Add the celery and carrot, mix well, and cook for about 3 minutes. Stir in the garlic and cook for 2 more minutes.

4. Add the wine, stir, and let cook and reduce for about 3 minutes. Add the tomato purée, heavy whipping cream, and beef stock, and mix well.

5. Partially cover and simmer for 4 hours, stirring often to prevent the sauce from sticking to the bottom. If you want it to be a little thicker, remove the lid for the last 30 minutes. It may make a mess as it simmers.

6. Taste and add salt and pepper to your liking.

Nutrition per Serving
206 calories | 14g fat | 15g protein | 5g carbohydrate | 1g fiber | 4g net carbohydrate

Resources

I want you to succeed, and I don't want to reinvent the wheel. There are already many fantastic resources in the world to support you in following all the recommendations I've made in this book. You'll find all my pro-tips in this chapter to help you skip over the pitfalls of a ketogenic diet and lifestyle change. If you're the type interested in reading everything you can about a topic, I'll be making many book recommendations, as well. I've got love for the other forms of useful media, too. There will be apps and websites and podcasts, oh my!

The resources and tips in this book are not exhaustive, and if you find something that speaks to you in ways that this book or the resources on this list have not, embrace it. Information is hardly ever enough to produce a change in our lives. It must be the right information, presented at the right time, in a way that speaks to us personally. Thankfully, today, there are many flavors of just about everything, information included.

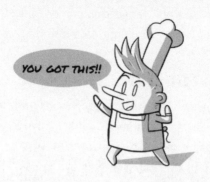

YOU GOT THIS!!

Ketogenic Diet Tips

The tips I've got for you (aside from the ones I gave you in the chapters) focus on two categories: eating out and social situations.

Eating Out

Though more and more restaurants are offering easy-to-identify keto friendly options, it can still be a challenge. In general, you can find something to eat at almost any restaurant if you are willing to ask the right questions, but there are still some places you will just have to skip.

At most places, the questions you need to ask are: Is there sugar or flour in the sauce? Is this breaded? Is the dressing made with sugar? Does the soup have flour or cornstarch? These are common sources of carbohydrates that are hidden in restaurant foods. Most service staff will not mind finding the answers, as long as you are polite when you ask.

Café-style restaurants may only have baked goods on their menus, which you will just have to skip. If you're really in a pinch and feel like you need some calories, just order coffee and put a lot of heavy whipping cream in there.

Social Situations

In America, every-dang thing revolves around food and often dessert-style food. Birthdays, holidays, baby showers, and meetings all offer cake, pie, scones, or muffins.

Avoiding carbohydrates can sometimes lead to awkward or exhausting conversations in which well-meaning people tell you that you are going to make yourself unhealthy with a diet that high in fat, or "just a little won't hurt."

You can avoid these conversations with a little verbal acrobatics. Don't say "I'm doing a keto diet" or "That's not on my diet." I've found success by starting with just a "Thanks, but I'm going to pass," and if pushed, moving on to "I'm attempting to change my relationship with food. It looks delicious, but I know I won't feel very good after eating it." If they are still nagging you and it is starting to make you uncomfortable, try to frame it in terms of support: "I'm really tempted but am trying to make better choices and would really appreciate your support with this challenge."

In my experience, if you couch the discussion in terms of health desires and social support, people are more likely to lay off on the carbohydrate pressure. If you find it *really* hard to stick to your goals in these types of situations, either just don't go to them or schedule one of your carb breaks when you know you'll be tempted.

Ketogenic Diet Resources

Books

If you want to dig deeper into the ketogenic diet, there are several good books on the market worth reading.

The Art and Science of Low Carbohydrate Living, by Steve Phinney, MD and Jeff Volek, PhD, RD–This book was written by a dietitian and a physician with years of clinical experience treating real people and hundreds of scientific publications about the ketogenic diet between them. Both authors are leaders in the field of ketosis.

Good Calories, Bad Calories, by Gary Taubes–This is a thoroughly researched and compellingly written account of why we, as a society, were told to eat low-fat, high-carbohydrate diets, and why that recommendation was likely a mistake. The author was a science journalist for years before he started writing about nutrition. If you pick this one up and are hungry for more like it, check out Taubes' other works, *Why We Get Fat* and *The Case Against Sugar.*

Quick Keto Meals in 30 Minutes or Less, by Martina Slajerova–This cookbook is one that my family has personally used and loved. The author has also written several other keto cookbooks worth pursuing if you like the recipes in this one.

Websites

www.ruled.me–This website has a ton of fantastic recipes for the ketogenic diet and occasional infographics and articles that are always informative and well researched.

www.peterattiamd.com–Peter Attia, MD, is a physician who is obsessed with pushing the boundaries of human performance and resilience. He covers topics like ketosis, fat metabolism, and nutrition research. All his articles are deep-dives and absolutely worth the time.

www.reddit.com–Reddit is a very popular aggregation website where almost all the content is user submitted and, for the most part, user regulated. It has thousands of "subreddits," which are niche communities on the site. Various ketogenic subreddits worth exploring include /r/keto, for general keto and mostly weight-loss information; /r/ketogains, which is is geared toward building muscle; /r/ketosceince; /r/ketorecipies; /r/vegetarianketo, which is less active than some of the other subreddits; and /r/xxketo, which is specifically for women.

www.ketoconnect.net–This recipe-driven website is worth spending some time on, because although the people that run this website are not dietitians or doctors, they are enthusiastic and thorough. They do all sorts of self-experiments, keto product reviews, and a lot of documenting.

Apps

In the beginning, while you are still getting a feel for estimating carbohydrate content, you may want to use one of the general food tracking apps. If you are interested in tracking calories, these apps make it a lot easier. I personally like MyFitnessPal best.

MyFitnessPal–This app is easy to use, has a huge database of foods, and allows you to create recipes and calculate homemade foods. However, some of the nutrient database comes from user entry so those items may not be entirely accurate.

FatSecret—This app has a huge database of foods. The free version shows net carbohydrate, if you're into that. User-submitted data is highlighted. However, it is less easy to use and has a cluttered interface.

Cron-O-Meter—Easy to use, very customizable. However, it doesn't divide tracked data into meals but keeps a tally for a full day. Additionally, it can only do custom recipes on the website.

Podcasts

There are many podcasts with a keto bent of varying quality. The ones I've listed tend to have worthwhile discussions. Keep in mind that this is not an exhaustive list.

Keto Talk with Jimmy Moore and Will Cole, DC—Jimmy Moore is a best-selling author in the keto world and has been living the lifestyle for over a decade. Will Cole is a chiropractor and functional medicine practitioner. Together they discuss many topics helpful to those following a ketogenic diet, as well as interview guests in that space.

The Keto Diet Podcast—Leanne Vogel is a holistic nutritionist who owns the popular blog Healthful Pursuit. Her podcast is a great source of support and inspiration for those looking to make a sustained lifestyle change. I'm interviewed in episode #47!

2 Keto Dudes—This is hosted by two middle-aged men that fought off diabetes and metabolic syndrome using a keto-genic diet. They discuss topics around the keto lifestyle in an

approachable and unassuming way. It can be pretty funny and at times has a morning-radio show feel, without all the crass jokes.

Low-Carb Resources

Books

The Paleo Diet, by Loren Cordain—While I don't adhere to or agree with all the recommendations outlined in this book, there is a lot of overlap. It is a great place to start for the rationale of sticking to whole foods and limiting carbohydrate and grains.

Wired to Eat, by Robb Wolf—If you are interested in the neurological and biochemical rationale of this diet, check out this work on the evolutionary argument for a low-carbohydrate baseline.

Salt, Sugar, Fat, by Michael Moss—Moss, a journalist who covers the food industry, outlines how the food industry uses salt, sugar, and fat to make processed foods nearly irresistible to humans. If you don't think this topic is interesting in its own right, think of it as an in-depth argument for why we should limit these formulated-to-be-addictive foods.

Websites

www.marksdailyapple.com—Mark Sisson is a retired professional athlete with one of the best low-carb blogs around. He regularly addresses issues that are relevant to living a low-carb/minimally processed lifestyle, and the website almost always links to primary research.

www.chriskresser.com–Kresser consistently puts out high-quality, well-researched content that is worth your time.

www.nomnompaleo.com–Recipes galore!

Podcasts

Nourish Balance Thrive–You may recall the name Nourish Balance Thrive from earlier in this book, when reading about ketosis and keto cycling. Nourish Balance Thrive is a holistic health and performance company headed by Dr. Tommy Wood and Chris Kelly. The guests on this podcast cover all the topics I've covered in this book plus more.

The Drive–Peter Attia, MD, hosts this podcast covering topics like sleep, meditation, fasting, ketosis, and more.

Balanced Bites–The podcast of Diane Sanfilippo and Liz Wolfe, both authors in the low-carb world. It is very conversational and can be very funny at times.

Fasting Resources

Books

Jump Start Ketosis: Intermittent Fasting for Burning Fat and Losing Weight, by Kristen Mancinelli–Mancinelli is a registered dietitian and expert on fasting and ketosis. This book is a well-researched and practical guide to incorporating intermittent fasting into your daily life, written in a fantastic conversational tone.

The Circadian Code–This book is written by one of the primary researchers in the field of intermittent fasting, Satchin

Panda, PhD. It covers the science behind why we should be limiting the window in which we eat, as well as science of circadian rhythm overall.

Apps

Zero—This is the only useful app I've seen for fasting or intermittent fasting. It's basically a fancy timer with predefined and customizable fasting windows. I do not use any app for fasting assistance, but if you prefer having a visual reminder of your fasting window, have at it.

Physical Activity Resources

Books

Starting Strength, by Mark Rippetoe—No matter what type of resistance training you choose to incorporate into your routine, this book is a great place to start. It covers the basic barbell movements like deadlifts and squats very well, but more importantly, it wonderfully details muscle and movement physiology.

Stress Management Resources

Books

10 Percent Happier, by Dan Harris—This is mostly a memoir of Dan Harris, an ABC correspondent that used meditation to manage his anxiety and addictive personality. It is a great place to start if you want to approach meditation in a manageable way. It is a quick read and Harris is a very relatable narrator.

Wherever You Go, There You Are, by Jon Kabat-Zinn—This is one of the most popular books ever written on mindfulness meditation. The author changed the perception of meditation in the research community and paved the way for some serious scientific inquiry.

Waking Up, by Sam Harris—If you want a humanist and non-religious approach to spirituality, this is your book.

Apps

Apps can be very useful for meditation practice because they can help guide you through the process of the different types of meditation, and if you find guided meditation to be a good fit for you, they provide you access to hundreds of guided meditations. I have found most of the meditation apps to be more or less the same. The important difference is the guide's voice and particular method of explaining the practice. Here are some that I have tried and can recommend. I suggest just picking one to start with and go from there.

- 10 Percent Happier
- Calm
- Headspace
- Insight Timer
- Simply Being
- The Mindfulness App

Selected References

For a full list of references, visit www.robertsantosprowse. com/CKD/reference.

"Childhood Obesity Facts." Centers for Disease Control and Prevention. Updated January 29, 2018. https://www.cdc.gov/ healthyschools/obesity/facts.htm.

"Overweight and Obesity." Centers for Disease Control and Prevention. Updated September 17, 2018. https://www.cdc .gov/obesity/index.html.

"Overweight and Obesity Statistics." *National Institute of Diabetes and Digestive and Kidney Diseases*. August 2017. https://www.niddk.nih.gov/health-information/ health-statistics/overweight-obesity.

"Trans Fats from Ruminant Animals May Be Beneficial." Redorbit.com. September 8, 2011. https://www.redorbit.com/news/health/2608879/ trans-fats-from-ruminant-animals-may-be-beneficial.

American Diabetes Association. "Economic Costs of Diabetes in the US in 2017." *Diabetes Care* 41, no. 5 (2018): 917-928. doi:10.2337/dci18-0007.

Brouwer, Ingeborg, Anne Wanders, and Martijn Katan."Effect of Animal and Industrial Trans Fatty Acids on HDL and LDL Cholesterol Levels in Humans—A Quantitative Review." *Plos ONE* 5, no. 3 (2010): e9434. doi:10.1371/journal .pone.0009434.

Corfe B.M., C.J Harden, M. Bull, and I Garaiova. "The Multifactorial Interplay of Diet, the Microbiome and Appetite Control: Current Knowledge and Future Challenges." *The Proceedings of the Nutritional Society* 74, no. 3 (2015): 235-44. doi: 10.1017/S0029665114001670.

Davison, James, Colin Lickwar, and Lingyun Song, et al. "Microbiota Regulate Intestinal Epithelial Gene Expression by Suppressing the Transcription Factor Hepatocyte Nuclear Factor 4 Alpha." *Genome Research* 27, no. 7 (2017): 1195-1206. doi:10.1101/gr.220111.116.

Fernandez, M.L. "Rethinking Dietary Cholesterol." *Current Opinion in Clinical Nutrition and Metabolic Care* 15, no. 2 (2012): 117-21. doi: 10.1097/MCO.0b013e32834d2259.

Gerster, H. (2018). "Can Adults Adequately Convert Alpha-Linolenic Acid (18:3n-3) to Eicosapentaenoic Acid (20:5n-3) and Docosahexaenoic Acid (22:6n-3)?" *International Journal for Vitamin and Nutrition Research* 68, no. 3 (1998): 159-73. https://www.ncbi.nlm.nih.gov/pubmed/9637947.

Huffman, Jennifer and Eric Kossoff. "State of the Ketogenic Diet(s) in Epilepsy." *Current Neurology and Neuroscience Reports* 6, no. 4 (2006)": 332-340. doi:10.1007/ s11910-006-0027-6.

Jones, P.J. A.S. Pappu, and L. Hatcher, et al. "Dietary Cholesterol Feeding Suppresses Human Cholesterol

Synthesis Measured by Deuterium Incorporation and Urinary Mevalonic Acid Levels." *Arteriosclerosis, Thrombosis, and Vascular Biology* 16, no. 10 (1996): 1222–8. https://www.ncbi.nlm.nih.gov/pubmed/8857917.

Malhotra, Aseem, Rita Redberg, and Pascal Meier. "Saturated Fat Does Not Clog the Arteries: Coronary Heart Disease Is a Chronic Inflammatory Condition, the Risk of Which Can Be Effectively Reduced from Healthy Lifestyle Interventions." *British Journal of Sports Medicine* 51, no. 15 (2017): 1111–12. doi:10.1136/bjsports-2016-097285.

Malhotra, Aseem. "Saturated Fat Is Not the Major Issue." *BMJ* 347 (2013): f6340. doi:10.1136/bmj.f6340.

Martin, Clayton, Maria Milinsk, and Jesuí Visentainer, et al. "Trans Fatty Acid-Forming Processes in Foods: A Review." *Anais Da Academia Brasileira De Ciências* 79, no. 2 (2007): 343–350. doi:10.1590/s0001-37652007000200015.

Patterson, E., R. Wall, and G. Fitzgerald, et al. "Health Implications of High Dietary Omega-6 Polyunsaturated Fatty Acids." *Journal of Nutrition and Metabolism* (2012): 1–16. doi:10.1155/2012/539426.

PLOS. "Sugar Industry Withheld Evidence of Sucrose's Health Effects Nearly 50 Years Ago, Study Suggests." ScienceDaily. Novemvber 21, 2017. https://www.sciencedaily.com/releases/2017/11/171121155819.htm.

Rivière, Audrey, Marija Selak, and David Lantin, et al. "Bifidobacteria and Butyrate-Producing Colon Bacteria: Importance and Strategies for Their Stimulation in the Human Gut." *Frontiers in Microbiology* 7 (2016). doi:10.3389/fmicb.2016.00979.

Rose, W. "II. The Sequence of Events Leading to the Establishment of the Amino Acid Needs of Man." *American Journal of Public Health and the Nations Health* 58, no. 11

(1968): 2020–27. https://www.ncbi.nlm.nih.gov/pmc/articles/
PMC1229034.

Sarris, Jerome, Alan Logan, and Tasnime Akbaraly, et al.
"Nutritional Medicine as Mainstream in Psychiatry." *The
Lancet: Psychiatry* 2, no. 3 (2015): 271–274. doi:10.1016/
s2215-0366(14)00051-0.

Tavernise, Sabrina. "F.D.A. Sets 2018 Deadline to Rid Foods of
Trans Fats." *New York Times.* June 16, 2015. https://www
.nytimes.com/2015/06/17/health/fda-gives-food-industry-
three-years-eliminate-trans-fats.html.

Teicholz, Nina. "The Scientific Report Guiding The US
Dietary Guidelines: Is It Scientific?" *BMJ* 351 (2015): h4962.
doi:10.1136/bmj.h4962.

Trepanowski, John, and Richard Bloomer. "The Impact of
Religious Fasting on Human Health." *Nutrition Journal* 9, no.
1 (2010). doi:10.1186/1475-2891-9-57.

Zahid, A. "The Vermiform Appendix: Not a Useless Organ."
Journal of the College of Physicians and Surgeons—Pakistan
14, no. 4 (2004): 256-8. doi: 04.2004/JCPSP.256258.

Index

Acknowledgments

I would like to acknowledge coffee.

I am also grateful to my wife and daughter for patiently accepting my absence during the many hours it took me to research and write this book. Geoff Pratt, the illustrator responsible for all of the images in this book, was a joy to work with and is one of my longest-standing conspirators. Thanks, pal.

Finally, I would like to thank the team at Ulysses Press for tolerating my perpetual disregard of deadlines and very sloppy submissions. Thank you, Shayna and Bridget!

About the Author

Robert Santos-Prowse is a registered dietitian and author. He specializes in low-carbohydrate and ketogenic diets and really likes broccoli. When not practicing clinical nutrition or writing, he can be found riding a bicycle or watching YouTube videos about science. If you ask him, he will absolutely tell you more than you want to know about the metabolic evils of a high-carbohydrate diet.

Learn more about him at www.robertsantosprowse.com.